INTRODUCE

BODY AND MIND
WITH
HOMOEOPATHY

By
Dr. Dipak Chakraborty

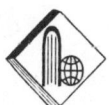

B. Jain Publishers Pvt. Ltd.
New Delhi

BODY AND MIND WITH HOMOEOPATHY

First Edition: 2000
3rd Impression: 2014

All rights reserved. No part of this book may be reproduced, stored in a retrieval system or transmitted, in any form or by any means, mechanical, photocopying, recording or otherwise, without any prior written permission of the publisher.

© with the Publisher

Published by Kuldeep Jain for
B. JAIN PUBLISHERS (P) LTD.
1921/10, Chuna Mandi, Paharganj, New Delhi 110 055 (INDIA)
Tel.: +91-11-4567 1000   Fax: +91-11-4567 1010
Email: info@bjain.com   Website: **www.bjain.com**

Printed in India

ISBN: 978-81-319-0672-9

DEDICATED TO

REVERED

MOTHER

Smt. Shyama Chakraborty

ACKNOWLEDGEMENT

I sincerely record my indebtedness to Dr.T.C. Bardoloi (New Delhi), Dr. M.K. Chakraborty (New Delhi), Dr. A.R. Mondal (Calcutta) for their valuable comments on the utility of the book.

I am grateful to Shri R.N. Das, M.A. BL, 411, R.K. Puram Sec 4, New Delhi who inspired me to a great extent and often enquired about the progress of the book.

I have much pleasure in expressing my gratitude and thanks to Dr. Bhavani Prasad Sahoo (recipient of Rabindranath Tagore Memorial Award), C N 134 DPL Township, Durgapur (WB), Dr.A.R. Bandyopadhyay, Medical Research Institute, Calcutta, Dr. Ratna Dey, Sr. Lecturer CMDE, Udharbond, Silchar (Assam), Dr. Tilak Bora, Margherita (Assam), Prof. Jayanta Chakraborty, Margherita (Assam) for their inspiration.

I should also express sincere thanks to Shri Manik Bhattacharjee, Kalibari Road, Dimapur (Nagaland) Shri Lakshman Gavender, NECL, Margherita (Assam), Shri Ashok Kumar Biswas, Immigration Officer, IGIA, New Delhi, Shri Surendera Kumar Agnihotri "Panchavati" R-20, Vani Vihar, Uttam Nagar,New Delhi- 59. Shri Anil Sharma, 35 S.P.Marg, New Delhi, Shri Pradip Kumar Bajra, 368, Lodi Colony, New Delhi, Shri Ramesh Pandit, RZ 28/F, Indira Park, Palam Colony, New Delhi, Shri Malay Som Choudhury, 12A, Banamali Chatterjee St., Calcutta-2, Shri Satish Sharma, Munirka, New Delhi, Shri Raju Mukherjee, 242 Dum Dum Park, Calcutta-55 and Miss Mahua Chakraborty,Carmel School, Digboi, Assam, for their inspiration and whole hearted co-operation in publication of this book.

( )

I must register a word of thanks and indebtedness to Shri Kuldeep Jain,1921 Chuna Mandi, Pahar Ganj, New Delhi 110055,without whose involvement this book could not have reached in your hands.

<u>*Dr. Dipak Chakraborty*</u>

Swami Pranavananda Homoeo Cure
Hospital Area,
P.O. Margherita,
Assam (786181)

FOREWORD

The sincere effort of Dr. Dipak Chakraborty, author of the book -**"Introduce Body & Mind with Homoeopathy"** is praiseworthy as he stressed on the need for life saving First Aid awareness.

In addition, this book represents a precise attempt for sharing knowledge on head to foot body mechanism and scopes for treatment of some common diseases under Homoeopathic system of medicines.

The book deserves appreciation from health point of view.

Dr. T.C. BARDOLOI
Addl. Deputy Director General
Directorate General of Health Services
Nirman Bhawan, New Delhi.11

FOREWORD

Dr. Dipak Chakraborty is to be congratulated on his commendable efforts for sharing knowledge on human body system, appeal for first aid conciousness and providing guide lines for treatment of various ailments under Homoeopathic system of medicines through the book- **"Introduce Body and Mind with Homoeopathy"**.

Hope, the health concious people in general will be benefited with this book which is probably first of its kind.

Dr. M.K. CHAKRABORTY
MBBS, DPH (Cal)
Addl. Medical Supdt.
Safdarjung Hospital
New Delhi -29.

FOREWORD

This is an age of 'progress' and 'readjustment' in medicine with many of our most cherished concepts of the past abandoned in the face of recent observations and experiments. The old order has changed. There is an increasing demand on the part of the overburdened to the society for the guidance of practical value in the daily pursuance of Health and medical practice.

Dr. D. Chakraborty's **"Introduce Body & Mind with Homoeopathy"** book should go a long way towards satisfying the demand of "Health For All".

I hope, this will provide a great help to the society.

Dr. A.R. MONDAL
MBBS, DCMS, DMS,DMSB (HONS)
Jt. Secretary, Homoeopathic Cancer & Aids Research Institute,
Life member,Indian Science Congress,
Asst.Doctor to Dr. B.N.Chakraborty.

INTRODUCTION

An attempt has been made to draw the attention of the persons who presume to know everything around the world but are ignorant about the mechanism in their own bodies. It may not be out of place to mention here that a good number of people are in the habit of self diagnosis and self medication and in doing so they sometimes fail to understand the Crux of the ailments. It has been noticed that some persons, being worried with various ailments, have approached the physicians in right manner but could not express their real problems merely due to their ignorance about the body organs. Moreover, misrepresentation of the facts does not help the doctors to proceed on the right track of investigation.

A few years back, a person came to me for consultation. He declared himself to be a patient of "damaged kidney" and expressed his desire to get cured at any cost. After necessary discussions and examination, it could be ascertained that the person had been suffering from some common ailments caused due to enlargement of his liver. In fact, his imagination about the location of kidney had caused him great anxiety. However, after necessary treatment, the patient came round quickly. I remember another such case in which a lady who had been suffering from urinary trouble since a long period, came to me for further consultation and casually expressed her concern over the death of her maternal uncle. She added that her uncle was suffering from 'Prostate' related illness and died within six months after detection. With a pale face, she wanted to know whether her urinary problems were related with Prostate. However considering her ignorance and growing fear of death, I vividly explained her about the role of Prostate Gland in a male body. She could understand that Prostate gland does not exist in a female body.

It is needless to tell the tales of ignorant people but it is wise to search for remedy. Keeping this in view, a sincere effort has been made to share the knowledge of human body system and functions of important organs and limbs, utility of First Aid, necessity of Vitamins and Minerals and other health guide lines through this book. The readers will also be advantageous to know about the scope for treatment of various diseases under Homoeopathy system of medicine.

Homoeopathy is an alternative system to cure the ailment of the suffering humanity. Dr.Samuel Fredericke Hahnemann of Miessen town in Germany who was a senior surgeon in Dresden Hospital of Modern Medicines (Allopathic) invented Homoeopathy in 1790 A.D. The therapeutic principle of Homoeopathy is - "Similia Similibus Curantur" i.e. diseases are treated with the medicines which are having capacity to produce symptoms of similar disease. In this system, the medicines are selected on the basis of the well marked symptoms, ideosyncracy of patients and drugs.

The word "treatment" in Medical Jargon is nothing but a war against the disease. The victory cannot be possible without a thorough observation on the enemy concentration as well as by way of using a particular weapon (vintage or sophisticated), tact and strategy. Similarly, with the purpose to fight against a disease, the medicine acts as weapon, diagnosis as an art and selection of proper medicine stands for strategy. Only with this understanding, success (cure) may be possible, if we can bridge the old, new and modern systems of medicines without giving scope for controversies over various systems of medicine. A scientific mind is ready to accept any conception - old or new.

My efforts will not go in vain, if the readers are benefited.

AUTHOR

Contents

FIRST AID	1
SKIN	17
HEAD	23
FACE	30
EYE	35
EAR	43
NOSE	47
LIPS	50
MOUTH	53
TOOTH	55
TONGUE	61
THROAT	65
HAND	73
CHEST	80
ABDOMEN	91
URINARY SYSTEM	102
LEGS	111
HEALTH GUIDE	117
VITAMINS	121
MINERALS	122
HEIGHT/ WEIGHT GUIDE	123
AN AVERAGE COMPOSITION OF BALANCED DIET	124
DIET LIMIT FOR DIABETICS	125

> **Note**
>
> *Any information given in this book is not intended to be taken as a replacement for medical advice. Any person with a condition requiring medical attention should consult a qualified practitioner or therapist.*

FIRST AID

A proper management and quick arrangement for First Aid are the twin major attempts to save a life from impending danger due to casualities like sudden injuries, bleeding (Haemorrhage), bone fracture, burn injuries, drowning, electrocution, food poisoning, choking (Block in Airways), heart attack, cerebral congestion, drug abuse, animal or insect bite, epilepsy etc.

For emergent use, a First Aid kit with the following assessories and medicines should be kept handy which may help cure and reduce risk. Besides, **First Aid awareness** with the knowledge of management is absolutely necessary for all the grown-up members of the family. For first aid awareness, a periodical discussion/questionnaire among the family members may be beneficial. Any active person with courage and knowledge of First Aid may save a life.

ASSESSORIES

1. One container or small box for keeping the medicines/assessories, preferably fitted with lock and key to avoid unnecessary handling or uncleaned touch.
2. One piece of unused Blade.
3. A pair of Scissors.

Where there is life, there is hope.

4. Artery Forceps.
5. One Cotton Roll.
6. One Bandage Roll.
7. Few pieces of Band-Aid.
8. Some pieces of cotton ribbon for use as rope.

MEDICINES :
- ARNICA MONTANA Q 1 oz.
- CALENDULA   Q 1 oz.
- HYPERICUM   Q 1 oz.
- CANTHARIS OINTMENT 1 tube
- APIS MEL.   30 1 dr. (Liquid)

The following methods of First Aid may be applied immediately to minimize the risk as and when threatened due to the conditions mentioned below:

1. BLEEDING : (Haemorrhage) : The human body contains 5 Litres. of Blood for maintaining circulatory system. Profuse bleeding or continuous bleeding may cause death.

In such conditions, the First Aid should be considered as Fast Aid without delay or waiting for a doctor. During emergency and when medicines or assessories are not available, the commonly used articles like shoe laces, hair ribbon, brief cases, school bags, scales, cloth pieces etc. may be pressed into service without hesitation.

The injured person should be taken to a well ventilated place and the bleeding part be cleaned with cold water first and then efforts should be made to obstruct the blood flow by pressing with fingers or palm.

In case of bleeding from lower extremities, the injured part should be drawn up form the body level of

Prevention is better than Cure.

First Aid

the victim. If possible, necessary support under the lifted part with available articles will be comfortable to the victim.

In case of bleeding from the upper extremities, the injured part should be drawn above the head of the victim. While bleeding is profuse, efforts should be made to tie the muscle 1 or 2 inches above the injured part. In emergent cases, available shoe laces, hair ribbon, pieces of plastic carry bags, pieces of cloth may be used without delay.

In case of bleeding due to detachment of limbs like fingers, hand, leg, toe, the injured part should be drawn up and tightly rolled with available cloth pieces, ribbon etc. The detached part should be picked up without hesitation or prejudice. Because, the detached part may be implanted by the expert surgeons. The victim should be rushed to the nearest hospital along with the detached limb.

While sharp or pointed substances are found in contact with the body and causes bleeding, such substances should never be removed till medical aid is available. Because, such substances remain as a pack in the bleeding part. Hence careless withdrawal of such substances may cause further injury and severe bleeding from the open wounds.

In case of profuse bleeding due to injury in head, back, chest, abdomen, the flow of blood may be obstructed by pressing with the palm or thumb on the injured part.

When the bleeding person is found in a conscious state, the victim should make effort himself to seal the wound by pressing the muscular part of hand, thigh or palm which can reach comfortably to the wound. The methods of First Aid should be continued till arrival of the doctor or hospitalisation.

Donate blood and save a life.

Nasal bleeding (Epistaxis) can be checked by keeping the hands straight above the head for few minutes. Gum-bleeding can be arrested by flossing with chilled water for few times.

2. BONE FRACTURE : There is a frame work of 206 bones in human body. The First Aid in Skull bone fracture and Spinal injury is difficult. In such conditions, the patient should be removed to the nearby hospital promptly and very carefully avoiding jerks.

In case of hand or leg bone fracture, no attempt should be made for setting the bone by pulling or pressing. Such attempt may cause further crack and other deformities. A cold compress with water or ice is beneficial. However, efforts should be made to provide a support below the fractured part with the help of a piece of wood or bamboo stick or scale whatever is available and tie up gently with cloth or laces before shifting to the nearby hospital.

Due to depletion of Calcium and other minerals, bone fracture may cause to the old people very easily in case of accident or fall. Due to hormone deficiency after menopause, bone fractures may cause to the ladies even due to minor reasons.

However, in case of dislocation, injury or fracture of bone, the patient should be removed to the hospital carefully as the detection can't be possible without X-Ray picture.

3. BURN : The burn injuries are very much common due to spread of fire in wearings or in uncovered skin. Careless handling of inflammable substances, bomb explosion, crackers and other fire works, electric shock, fall of boiling water or milk etc. The body may sustain injuries affecting skin, tissues, to a maximum degree. Any

---

Neglegency carry risk.

type of burn, causes restless condition due to severe burning, pain, fear, anxiety etc. In some cases, the victim may fall unconscious. In case of fire spreads on the wearings of a person, a wet bed-sheet/blanket or any other clothings should immediately be wrapped over the entire body of the victim. The victim should never be allowed to run or rest near a moving fan till fire is estinguished. When water or cloth sheets are not available, all efforts should be made to put off or tear out the wearings. Flushes of cold water or application of coconut oil over the burn injury reduces burning sensation, pain etc. Application of mud or crushed potatoes also reduces the blisters and pain.

When the victim is found in restless condition or unconscious state with severe burn, efforts should be made for immediate hospitalisation, Ensure proper ventilation till the victim is brought to the hospital.

In case of minor burn injuries, application of cold compress is to be continued for a longer period.

4. DROWNING : Immediately after rescue, the first attempt is absolutely necessary to drain out water from the victim's stomach. It can be possible by placing the victim's abdomen on a supporting barrel or cylindrical article or on the back of any person (in animal position being supported on knees and hands on the ground). In this position, the victim's head and legs will be placed below the abdomen level naturally. A rhythmic pressure on the victim's abdomen from opposite side (back side) is necessary to drain out water from the stomach.

After drainage of water, the victim is to be shifted to a normal lying position for providing mouth to mouth breathing (respiration). The Carotid Artery pulsation is to be checked time to time to asses the response of the artificial respiration (see page 9). Necessary arrangement should be made for immediate hospitalization.

5. ELECTROCUTION : Electric shock may cause severe burn and death in no time. All efforts should be made promptly to rescue the victim. The rescuer must follow the caution given below :

1. Do not touch the person got eletrocuted.
2. Switch off the main line immediately.
3. Do not act bare-footed.
4. Do not apply any wet object.
5. Do not apply any metallic objects.
6. Do not apply raw or wet bamboo sticks.
7. Raise hue and cry for help.

In case the power line could not be disconnected, a direct hit (Strike) with a dry piece of wood or back of a wooden chair aiming at the contact area may help rescue of the victim. Immediately after the rescue, a thorough massage on the victim's entire body is a must to remove circulatory obstructions. As and when necessary, artificial respiration (see page 9) should be given promptly and continued till medical assistance is available.

6. FOOD POISONING : Commonly it causes obstinate vomiting, diarrhoea, bloated abdomen, restless condition, dehydration, and respiratory trouble. In such conditions, the body fluid is to be maintained (Rehydration) by providing clean and cold water mixed with a little salt and sugar at frequent intervals till medical treatment is available.

Donate blood and save a life.

First Aid

When a person consumes poison deliberately or unknowingly, efforts should be made for immediate hospitalization. Because, the condition of the patient may turn critical if the stomach is not cleaned (Suction) immediately. The suction may not be possible without hospitalization.

7. CHOKING : The throat is the gate-way for air and food. Due to unmindful eating, sudden fear, tension, any solid food may get stuck in the throat. In such cases breathing is not possible due to block in the trachea (air-way). This condition may cause death even, but only a prompt First Aid may save the life.

Boost up the morale of the patient and make him stand up and mouth open. Ask the patient to keep his head in normal position. The rescuer must take his position behind the victim and hit heavily on the upper back (between shoulder blades) with fist. Repeat the method 4/5 times rapidly. If this method fails to clear the block, hold the victim's abdomen clutching the fingers of both the hands just above the umbilical area (Navel) and press the stomach with great force. Continue this method till the release of the foreign body. If there is none to help, the victim himself may apply this method by placing his own abdomen on the back of a sofa, chair or side of any bed.

If the victim becomes air hunger, mouth to mouth artificial breathing (see page 9) should be given till medical aid is available.

When any foreign body gets stuck in the airways of an infant, make the victim lie on front and upside down and hit on the back (between shoulder blades) with fist carefully.

Today's Neglegency: Tomorrows Repentation.

Remember, all efforts should be made to clear the air ways **within 3 minutes** i.e. 180 seconds. Otherwise the condition of the victim may turn critical, leading to death.

8. HEART ATTACK : It may cause due to high blood pressure (Hypertension), shock, stress, high cholesterol level, diabetic condition etc. Sudden palpitation of heart, severe chest pain, fainting, profuse sweating are common signs of heart attack.

In such cases, make loose the clothings of the paient and ensure proper ventilation. In no case water should be given to drink. It may cause plug in the throat and deterioration of the patient's condition.

Place the patient on a bench, cot or table to ensure a hard bed (lying on a hard surface) keeping the body straight. Do not give pillow under the head. Watch the pulse nearer to the wrist (thumb side). Pulsation may be rapid, slow or absent. Raise the lower side of the cot (foot side) at least 18 inches above by placing anything like bricks, bundle of newspaper or folded bed roll, whatever is available immediately. When the patient is on the ground, his/her legs are to be drawn 18 inches up by giving a support. In this process, the victim's head and upper extremities will get supply of blood due to gravitation from lower extremities. Then try for opening the mouth of the victim. Because, accumulation of saliva, sticky fluid, food stuff etc. inside the mouth or throat may obstruct breathing. So clean the mouth and throat by applying two fingers (indicator and middle finger) at a time or with the help of a rolled cloth piece. To keep the airways wide open, lift the victim's chin and keep parallel to the chest. It can be done by lifting the victim's neck and a backward pressure on the forehead carefully. Take only 30 seconds for bringing the victim's body in a correct position up to this level.

Prevention is better than cure.

First Aid

Now the position is ready for **Cardiac Massage and Artificial Respiration** (Mouth to mouth or mouth to nose breathing).

Watch the breathing condition of the patient. This can be observed by putting ear nearer to the victim's nostrils. Otherwise put a spect near the nostrils of the patient. The glass will get vaporized when breathing is present.

Watch the pulse of the victim. If pulsation is absent near the wrist, place the thumb and indicator spreading over the Carotid arteries on the neck. When pulsation is absent, consider it to be a case of heart attack or cardiac respiratory failure. In such cases, the following methods of First Aid may be adopted immediately to save the victim.

(A) ARTIFICIAL RESPIRATION (Mouth to mouth or mouth to nose breathing.)

When the pulse is found slow or absent, clip the nostrils of the patient with thumb and first finger (indicator). Inhale lungful air. Place your mouth on the victim's mouth and blow air with great force. Ensure expansion (rise) of victim's chest while giving artificial breathing. If the mouth is not properly sealed with victim's mouth, the air may not rush inside the victim's lungs. For safety reasons, check the victim's teeth and remove denture if any, before giving artificial respiration.

When the victim's mouth is found closed, the artificial respiration should be given through the nostrils. Seal the victim's mouth by placing the palm before giving respiration through the nostrils.

Artificial respiration should be given 2 times at an interval of 5 seconds and switch over to cardiac massage.

Smoking is injurious to health.

(B) CARDIAC MASSAGE : This is another method for stimulating the Heart.

Place your palm on the reverse side of another palm clutching the fingers. Keep the hands straight and steady. Place the **heel of the palm** (Picture 1) on the centre of the victim's chest in a parallel position with both the nipples. This is the location of a flat bone called **Sternum**, suppose to be a guard protecting the human heart. Due to a particular shape, size and location, the Sternum can bear maximum pressure. So the heart may be pumped artificially by giving rhythmic pressure (compression) on the **Sternum**.(Picture 2)

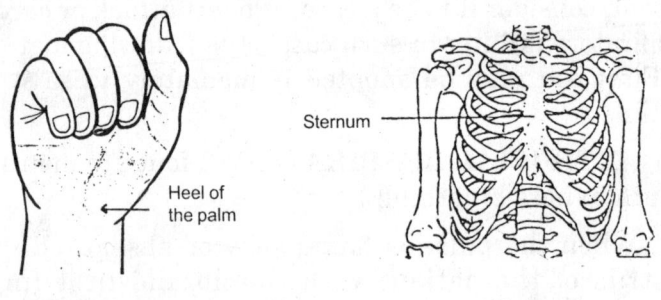

Picture-1   Picture-2

After providing artificial respiration twice, give 15 compressions within 15 seconds. Continue both the methods alternately as ratio given below:

Artificial respiration   : 2 times (Five seconds interval)
Compression   : 15 times   (per second 1 compression)

All efforts should be made within 3 minutes to save a dying person.

It may be mentioned here that in case of children or infants, the compression should be given carefully only

Negligency carry risk.

with two fingers instead of heel of the palm. However, the Cardiac Massage should be stopped after restoration of the pulse. Otherwise, the afore said methods should be continued till the medical aid is available.

9. ANIMAL/INSECT BITE : In case of dog or other animal bite, flush the wound with cold water for a long time. It is advisable to use speedy water flow directly from a tap or other sources for cleaning the wound and surrounding parts. This is the best way to minimise the risk. After cleaning for a long time, cover the wound with a cotton cloth piece and rush for medical treatment.

In case of snake, scorpion, spider bite, it is advisable to obstruct blood circulation immediately with the help of tight bandages on the parts above and below the bite spot (Picture 3).

Picture-3

From practical experience, the following medicines under Homoeopathic System have been shown to be very effective for emergent treatment with recommended doses as mentioned against the ailments.

Food Poisoning : **Arsenic Alb. 30**
1 drop with half spoon cold water 6 times at 5 mnts. interval.

Safety first.

Heart Attack with Chest Pain.	: **Agaricus 30** 1 drop with half spoon cold water 5 times at 5 mnts. interval.
Cerebral Congestion	: **Aconite Nap. 30** 3 drops with 1 spoonful cold water 4 times at 10 mnts. interval
Eye ball injury	: **Symphytum 30** 1 drop with half spoon cold water half hourly 4 times a day.
Eye injury	: **Ruta G. 200** 1 drop with a spoonful cold water 1 hourly 4 times a day.
Injury from Nail, Iron, Blade etc.	: **Ledum Pal. 1x** To be applied locally. **Ledum Pal. 30** 1 drop with half spoon cold water 4 times at 10 mnts. interval.
Badly shocked due to injury or fall.	: **Aconite Nap. 30** 4 drops on tongue directly 4 times at 10 mnts. interval.
Clean wounds	: **Staphisagria 30** 1 drop with half spoon cold water 4 times at 15 mnts. interval.
Torn wounds	: **Calendula 30** 1 drop with half spoon cold water 5 times at 15 mnts. interval.

Person lacking of humanitarian act is unsocial.

First Aid

Punctured Wounds	: **Ledum Pal. 30** 1 drop with half spoon cold water 4 times at 5 mnts. interval.
Lacerated Wounds	: **Hamamelis V. Q** To be applied locally.
	: **Hamamelis 30** 1 drop with half spoon cold water 4 times at 15 mnts. interval daily. Continue for 3 days.
Lock-jaw	: **Hypericum 30** 1 drop with half spoon cold water 4 times at 10 mnts. interval daily.
Injury from Bomb Blast	: **Calendula Q** To be applied locally. **Aconite Nap. 30** 1 drop with half spoon cold water 4 times at 5 mnts. interval.
Battle injury	: **Hypericum Q** To be applied locally. **Arnica Mont. 30** 1 drop with half spoon cold water 5 times at 5 mnts. interval.
Bullet injury	: **Hypericum Q** To be applied locally **Aconite Nap. 30** 3 drops with half spoon cold water 5 times at 10 mnts. interval.

Donate blood and save a life.

Shooting pain in injured part	: **Hypericum Q** 3 drops with 2 tea spoonful cold water 4 times at 15 mnts. interval.
Nose Bleed (Epistaxis)	: **Milllefolium Q** 5 drops with 2 spoon-full cold water 1 hourly 3 times.
Bleeding from orifice of the body	: **Hamamellis Vir. 30** 1 drop with half spoon cold water 4 times at 10mnts. interval.
Blood Vomiting	: **Ferr. acct. 30** 1drop with half spoon cold water 4 times at 10 mnts. interval.
Blood with coughing	: **Ipecac 30** 1 drop with half spoon cold water 5 times at 5 mnts. interval.
Gum Bleeding	: **Acid Nitricum 30** 2 drops with half spoon cold water 4 times at 15 mnts. interval.
Blood with Urine	: **Cantharis 3x** 3 drops with 1 spoonful cold water 4 times at 15 mnts. interval.
Rectal Bleeding	: **Acid Nitricum 6** 3 drops with 1 spoonful cold water 4 times at 10 mnts. interval.

Donate eye and let see others.

First Aid

Uterine Bleeding	: **Phosphorus 30** 1 drop with half spoon cold water 5 times at 10 mnts. interval with bed rest.
Profuse Bleeding after delivery.	: **Cinemonon Q** 5 drops with 4 spoonful cold water half hourly 3 times with bed rest.
Burns	: **Cantharis Ointment.** To be applied locally. **Cantharis 30** 2 drops with half spoon cold water 5 times at 10 mnts. interval.
Burns with pain	: **Urtica. Urens 30** 1 drop with half spoon cold water 4 times at 5 mnts. interval.
Bone injury	: **Symphytum 30** 2 drops with 1 spoonful cold water 3 hourly 4 times daily for 4 days.
Spinal injury	: **Hypericum 30** 1 drop with half spoon cold water 4 times at 15 mnts. interval daily for 3 days.
Bite	: **Ledum 30** 1 drop with half spoon cold water 4 times at 5 mnts. interval.

Donate blood and save a life.

Rabit Bite	: **Hypericum Q** To be applied locally, and 4 drops with 2 spoonful cold water 2 hourly 3 times.(oral)
Scorpion Bite	: **Calotropis Gigantia Q** 5 drops with 2 tea spoonful cold water 2 hourly 3 times.

■■

SKIN

The skin is a surface layer of tissue covering from head to foot. Due to its co-ordinating function with brain and spinal cord, the skin is one of the sensasory organs with prime role in the body. Because of the spread nerve endings, the skin is very much sensitive to touch and environmental temparature. The skin is the chief organ to maintain body temparature by dissipating heat to the surrounding air and protect body from dehydration or any kind of pathogenic organisms and their toxin by its defending mechanism. But the skin is more vulnerable during the period of childhood and pregnancy. The skin consists of **Epidermis, Dermis and Subcuteneous** layers.

The surface layer with only epithelial cells is Epidermis. Epithelium is the main tissue of the outer layer of the skin which can produce daughter cells immediately for natural repairing of any wear and tear condition of skin. The pores of the epidermis are the outlets of perspiration and oil from sweat glands.

There are no blood vessels in epidermis, but the living cells in its deepest layer produce **'Melanin'**, the pigment that gives skin its colour but purely depends on dermis for nourishment.

Cleanliness is heavenliness.

The inner layer with a frame work of connective tissues, blood vessels, nerve endings and oil glands is Dermis which rests upon the Subcutaneous layer.

The Subcuteneous layer of the skin contains part of glands, fat deposits to regulate energy. It also contains skin appendages like hair and nails. The **elastic collagen fibres** provide support from underneath.

The thickness of the epidermis and dermis varies in some parts of body like eye lids, palms and soles.

Exposure to strong tropical sunlight or heat, increase the flow of 'Melanin' from epidermis which may lead to discolourisation of skin. Moreover, deffient supply of Vitamins may develop problems like dehydration, scalling, scabbies, eczema, boils, black pores, urticaria or other allergic erruption. Worms may also aggravate skin trouble. Mental stress may also lead to skin disorders like puffiness, dark shadows, fine lines etc. smoking habit also ages skin prematurely. Due to staphylococcus aureus, unhygienic environment or cross infection, skin diseases like **Pemphigus Neonatorum, Septicaemia or Pyaemia** some times found in new born babies. Such diseases are usually associated with systematic illness including fever and erruption of blisters, pustules on the palms, soles and trunk. In such cases, consultation with a child specialist should not be delayed.

In case of any contegious erruption, appearance of white spots or abnormal skin colour, it is suggested to consult Dermatologist as early as possible. Moderate food habit, cleanliness and hygenic wearings should be given priority for healthy skin. Intake of cold water sufficiently is necessary for skin smoothness.

Natural Food is Vital Food.

Skin

A Balanced Diet including the following Vitamins, Proteins and Minerals is absolutely necessary for maintenance of skin.

Vitamins :   A -   Butter, Buttermilk, Curd, Eggs, Sweet Potatoes, Carrots, Papaya, Mango, Green Vegetables.

B2-   Peas, Green Vegetables.

C-   Oranges, Sweet lime, Gooseberrie (Amla), Lemon, Strawberries, Guava, Tomatoes. Corriander, Germinated pulses/gram, Potatoes, green leafy vegetables.

D-   Cod-liver oil, Fatty fish, Liver, Butter and the sources from Sunlight.

E-   Dal, Rice, Eggs etc.

Protein :   Pulses, Nuts, Dry fruits, Fish, Milk, Meat, Eggs.

Minerals :

Sodium / Potassium -   Salt, Most foods, green Coconut water.

The sunrays are very strong when the shadow is shorter than the subject and moderate when the shadow is taller than the subject. Strong Sunrays should be avoided.

However, the following Homoeopathic medicines have been shown to be effective for healing of some common ailments of the skin.

Prevention is better than cure.

Skin

Unhealthy Skin	: **Calcarea Carb. 6** 2 drops with half spoon cold water 3 hourly 4 times daily for 7 days.
Bad smell (odour) from body	: **Sulphur 200** 1 drop with 1 spoon cold water once daily for 3 days.
Burning sensation in skin	: **Cantharis 200** 1 drop with 1 spoon cold water once daily for 5 days
Erruption due to secondary syphilis	: **Merc. Cor. 30** 2 drops with 1 spoon cold water 3 hourly 4 times daily for 7 days.
Insensibility of skin	: **Opium 200** 1 drop with 1 spoonful cold water once daily for 7 days.
Boils all over the body	: **Arnica Montana 200** 2 drops with 1 spoonful cold water 3 hourly 4 times daily for 3 days.
Warts (Masa)	: **Thuja 200** 1 drop with half spoon cold water once daily for 10 days.
Vesicles on skin	: **Cantharis 200** 1 drop with half spoon cold water 3 hourly 4 times daily for 3 days.
Tendency to Gangrene	: **Carbo Veg. 200** 1 drop with half spoon cold water 3 hourly 2 times daily for 7 days.

Frequent exposure to X-Ray is injurious to health.

Skin

Sweating at night	: **Calcarea Carb. 30** 2 drops with half spoon cold water 3 hourly 3 times daily for 5 days.
Foul smell from sweating parts	: **Plumbum 200** : 1 drop with half spoon cold water once daily for 7 days.
Ringworm	: **Baccilinum 200** 1 drop with half spoon cold water 3 hourly 3 times daily for 3 days.
Obstinate ringworm	: **Jelluricum 6** 2 drops with 1 spoonful cold water 3 hourly 3 times daily for 5 days.
Urticaria	: **Urtica Urens 30** 1 drop with half spoon cold water half hourly 3 times a day.
Allergy after taking Tomato	: **Lyco Persicum 30** 2 drops with 1 spoonful cold water once daily for 3 days.
Eczema on scalp	: **Petrolium 200** 1 drop with half spoon cold water 3 times daily for 3 days.
Eczema in scrotum	: **Croton Tinglium 6** 2 drops with 1 spoonful cold water 3 hourly 3 times daily for 7 days.
Any kind of skin erruption with itching severely	: **Petrolium 30** 2 drops with half spoon cold water itching severely 3 hourly 4 times for 2 days.

Neglegency carry Risk.

Itching with oedamatus swelling of skin.	: **Apis Mel. 30** : 2 drops with half spoon cold water 1 hourly 4 times daily for 2 days.
Itching in normal skin	: **Dolichos Prulicus 30** 2 drops with half spoon cold water 3 hourly 4 times a day.
Eczema do not heal rapidly	: **Calcarea Carb. 30** 2 drops with 1 spoonful cold water 3 hourly 4 times daily for 10 days.
Pustular boils	: **Hepar Sulphur 200** 1 drop with half spoon cold water 3 hourly 4 times daily for 2 days.
Carbancle	: **Tarentula Cubensis 200** 1 drops with half spoon cold water once daily for 7 days.
Sun stroke	: **Glonoin 30** 2 drops with half spoon cold water 3 hourly 4 times daily for 2 days.
Sudden painful sensitiveness of skin.	: **Coffea Cruda 30** 2 drops with half spoon cold water 1 hourly 4 times a day.

■■

Natural food is vital food.

HEAD

The skull of the head is composed of the following 8 Cranial bones called-Frontal Bone (1) Parietal Bones (2), Temporal Bones (2), Ethmoid Bone (1), Sphenoid Bone (1), Occiputal Bone (1).

Two types of muscles called **Temporalis** and **Frontalis** are there in the head.

The Head with a brain circuit is the control tower with multifarious signal system to regulate entire biological activities. For instance, the anterior temporal lobe regulates the sense of appetite, excretion and governs memory through visual, audio and physio-motor systems. Over exhaustion, shock, grief, emotion, fear, anger, jeolous nature, genetic influence, dehydration and mal-nutrition may lead to a stress situation which sets off a biological alarm in the brain circuit and causes irregularities in body chemistry.

Such irregularities may produce an immediate physical reaction which hastens the onset of various diseases like Diabetes Mellitus, Hypertension, Heart attack, Sleeplessness, Loss of appetite, Forgetfulness, Asthma and Headache of different sufferings including Migrane.

Your Mind can keep you active.

There is a saying - 'Your mind can keep you active'. It bears justification. Because, healing can't be possible without **Mind** and **Body** interactions. The habit of learning to think right, do right and to maintain the attitude always pleasant and cheerful as possible may be the only source to keep the body and mind fit. Better avoid controversy and challange in trifling matters to lead a peaceful, healthy and cheerful life.

To avoid mal-nutrition hazards, top priority should be given for a balanced diet (Chart on page no.124) including the essential Vitamins and Minerals which could be available from natural sources for nutrition of Brain and Hair as mentioned below :

Vitamins	:	A	: Spinach, Carrots, Sweet Potatoes Mango, Butter.
	:	B1	: Eggs, Meat, Whole Cereals.
	:	B12	: Fish, Pork.
Minerals	:	Iron	: Cereals,Pulses, Green vegetables Heeng.(Asafoetida)
		Magnesium	: Green leafy vegetables, Cereals
		Phosphorus	: Cereals,Pulses, Milk.
		Sulphur	: Cereals, Pulses.

It may not be out of place to highlight the problems relating to hair. Erruption on Scalp, dandruff, using variety of hair oil, shampoo, environmental pollution, stomach disorders, anaemia, typhoid, hormonal imbalance, sleeplessness, depletion of mineral salts are the major factors behind hair fall, early greying and

Head

baldness etc. Since, East-West hair style is much in vogue, the complaints like hair fall, baldness are undoubtedly alarming while mature or premature greying may not cause anxiety. Because, hair dying chemicals are being used as the most common item as an essential commodity. But it is not known whether such chemicals are free from side effects including interference in normal brain functioning or any impact on next generation.

However, some common ailments relating to head, brain and hair could be treated with the following Homoeopathic medicines with recommended doses.

Errupted scalp : **Mezerium 200**
1 drop with half spoon cold water 3 hourly 4 times daily for 2 days.

Hair fall : **Chionanthus Ix**
20 drops with half cup of cold water for application on scalp daily after bath for 15 days.

Suddenly appeared headache : **Belledonna 200**
1 drop on tongue directly 3 hourly 3 times a day.

Headache from exposure to cold : **Aconite Nap. 30**
2 drops with a spoonful cold water 1 hourly 3 times a day.

Headache with coldness of limbs : **Helleborus N. 30**
1 drop with half spoon cold water half hourly 4 times a day.

Inability to hold up head due to congestive headache : **Glonoine 30**
1 drop with half spoon cold water 4 times at 10 mnts. interval a day.

Good Health is the noblest gift of God.

Severe headache	: **Coffea Cruda 30** 1 drop with half spoon cold water 4 times at 10 mnts. interval a day.
Headache after a fall or injury	: **Arnica Mont 30** 1 drop with half spoon cold water 6 times at 15 mnts. interval for 2 days.
Headache after niddle work or eye strain.	: **Ruta G. 200** 1 drop with 1 spoon cold water 2 times at 20mnts. interval for a day.
Bruised pain in head while moving	: **Cuprum Met. 200** 1 drop with half spoon cold water half hourly 2 times a day.
Headache due to heat	: **Aconite Nap. 30** 2 drops with 1 spoon cold water half hourly 3 times a day.
Occiputal headache	: **Belladonna 200** 1 drop with half spoon cold water half hourly 3 times a day.
One sided headache	: **Pulsatilla 200** 1 drop with half spoon cold water half hourly 3 times a day.
Headache due to riding a car	: **Petrolium 200** 1 drop with a spoonful cold water 3 times at 20 mnts. interval.

Green Vegetable is essential for nutrition.

Head

Heaviness in forehead	: **Calcarea Carb. 30** 1 drop with half spoon cold water 3 times at 15 mnts. interval.
Cerebral congestion	: **Aconite Nap. 3x** 3 drops with a spoonful cold water 4 times at 10 mnts. interval.
Sleeplessness	: **Opium 200** 1 drop with half spoon cold water 1 hourly 2 times daily evening for 2 days.
Meningitis	: **Helleborus N. 200** 1 drop with half spoon cold water 1 hourly 3 times a day.
Noise upsets	: **Coffea Cruda 200** 1 drop with half spoon cold water 3 hourly 3 times a day.
Stiff Neck	: **Apis Mel 30** 1 drop with half spoon cold water half hourly 4 times a day.
Weak Memory	: **Brahmi Q** 5 drops with 1 spoonful cold water 2 times daily at morning and evening for 15 days.
Brain Fag	: **Picric Acid 30** 2 drops with 1 spoonful cold water 3 hourly 3 times daily for 7 days.

Keep Diet Balance.

Tone up memory	: **Argentinum Nitricum 200** 1 drop with 1 spoonful cold water once daily for 7 days.
Depression	: **Phosphoric Acid 30** 1 drop with 1 spoonful cold water 3 hourly 3 times daily for 2 days.
Mental imbalance	: **Platinum 200** 1 drop with half spoon cold water 3 hourly 3 times daily for 7 days.
Anxiety during Examination	: **Argentinum Nitricum 200** 1 drop with half spoon cold water 1 hourly 2 times daily during examination period.
Fear of death	: **Aconite Nap. 30** 2 drops with half spoon cold water 1 hourly 3 times daily for 3 days.
Anticipatory Fear	: **Lycopodium 200** 1 drop with 1 spoonful cold water 3 hourly 3 times daily for 3 days.
Suicidial tendency	: **Aurum Met. 30** 2 drops with 1 spoonful cold water 3 hourly 3 times daily for 3 days.
Delusion (Speaks linkless)	: **Cannabis Indica 30** 2 drops with half spoon cold water once daily morning for 10 days.

Strong Medicines Have Strong Reactions.

Head

Severe Convulsion	: **Cuprum Met. 30** 1 drop with half spoon cold water 4 times at 5 mnts. interval.
Sudden fainting	: **Amylium Nitrate Q** few drops in cotton for inhalation only.
Emotional fainting	: **Coffea Cruda 200** 1 drop with half spoon cold water half hourly 3 times.
Fainting due to fear, shock	: **Ignatia 200** 1 drop with half spoon cold water 1 hourly 3 times a day for 2 days.
Hysteria	: **Nux Moschata Q** 5 drops with 2 spoonful cold water 4 hourly 3 times daily for 2 days.
Fainting with snoaring breathing and face become dark	: **Opium 200** 1 drop with half spoon cold water 3 times at 10 mnts. interval.
Fainting with changes in skin colour	: **Glonoine 30** 1 drop with half spoon cold water 4 times at 5 mnts. interval during the attack. (Should be given with care).
Fainting with pressed teeth, foaming and bluish colour.	: **Acidum Hydro Sionic 30** 2 drops with one spoon cold water 3 times at 10 mnts. interval.
Fainting with redness in colour	: **Belladona 30.** 2 drops with half spoon cold water 4 times at 5 mnts. interval.

Health is Wealth, Preserve it.

FACE

The facial portion is composed of 14 bones including the following :

Mandible-1, **Maxillae**-2, **Zygomatic**-2, **Nasal Bones**-2, **Lacrimal bones**-2, **Vomer**-1, **Paletine bones** 2, **Inferior Nasal Conchae**-2.

The following are the facial muscles :

Orbicularis Oris, Orbicularis Oculi, Levator Palpabrae Superioris, Buccinator, Temporalis and masseter.

Face is the index of mind and body. Mental state like pleasure, depression, intelligentia, dullness, affection, lust, cruelty, fear-pshycosis, suppression of facts could be read easily on the face of a person. Moreover, sleeplessness eye strain, anaemia and other sickness also reflects on human faces.

Even during a special care for face, some problems like erruption of pimples/acene, sunburn, black pores, dark stains below the eyes, dry scalling of skin, perspiration, unwanted hair growth or delayed projection of maleness are very common due to biological changes, climatic changes and mal-nutrition.

Green vegetable is essential for nutrition.

Face

Erruption of pimples or acene is the most common threat to the facial skin. During adolescence, some physical and chemical changes occur in the body system. Sebaceous glands below the skin's surface produce small quantities of oily material known as Sebum. These glands stop secretion after 22 years of age.

When pores gets clogged due to dirt or excess secretion of Sebum, skin bacteria feast on oily material (Sebum) and gradually releases toxic stuff and inflame the pores. In some cases, immune system reacts at this stage resulting in erruption of pimples/acene on the forehead, cheeks and other uncovered parts of the body.

Commonly pimples are of two types. Some people suffers from painful erruption of pimples with a white dot (pus) in centre while others with a black dot. A sudden increase in erruption of pimples may be experienced during summer season due to hot exposure.

Frequent exposure to sun may cause damage to facial skin and develop hyper-pigmented brown or copper colour patches or dropsical swelling, wrinkles, fine lines. The ultra-violet radiation in sunlight breaks down the elastic collagen that supprot the skin. Sprinkling of cold water on face immediately after moving in sun during summer season may develop black pores on facial skin. Stress, sleeplessness (insomnia) and irregular bowels, run-down condition of health may develop dark circular patches below the eyes. Use of various cosmetics and periodical bleaching, hair dye, repeated use of soap on face, habit of smoking, intake of less water, defficiency of Vitamins and Minerals are the common factors behind dry scalling of facial skin.

Face is the index of mind.

The following guide lines are enough for make-up or protection of facial skin.

* Avoid direct sun light during summer season. Both dark or bright skins are vulnerable to sun burn.
* Avoid pricking of pimples with nails.
* Avoid regular use of cosmetics and bleaching.
* Avoid regular use of soap and rubbing of face.
* Washing of oily face with cold water.
* Intake of plenty water daily.
* Use black umbrella particularly in summer season.
* Taking of sufficient green vegetables and citrus fruits daily.
* A balanced diet with necessary nutrients as given below :

Vitamins- A		(Spinach, Carrots, Sweet Potatoes, Mangoes, Butter, Fish, Liver)
	B2	(Green leafy vegetables, Peas, Milk, Eggs, Liver).
	C	(Fresh fruits, Lemon, Banana, Oranges, Goose-berries ,Guava).
	D	(Liver, Fish, Cod Liver Oil, Milk, Butter).
Minerals-Iron		(Cereals, Pulses, Green vegetables, Banana, Cumin, Zeera, heeng, Meat).
	Sulphur	(Cereals, Pulses)
	Sodium/ Potassium	(Salt, most foods, coconut).

Good Health is the noblest gift of God.

Face

The following Homoeopathic medicines are found more effective for treatment of some common ailments relating to facial skin.

Sweating on face	:	**Calcarea Carb. 30** 2 drops with half spoon cold water once at daily morning for 10 days.
Pustules on face	:	**Merc. Cor. 30** 2 drops with half spoon cold water 3 hourly 4 times daily for 3 days.
Small painful pimples on face	:	**Arnica Montana 30** 2 drops with half spoon cold water 3 hourly 4 times daily for 3 days.
Vesicles on face	:	**Cantharis 200** 1 drop with half spoon cold water 3 hourly 4 times daily for 2 days.
Black pores on face	:	**Sulphur 30** 2 drops with a spoonful cold water 3 hourly 3 times daily for 7 days.
Dropsical swelling of face	:	**Apis Mel. 30** 2 drops with a spoonful cold water 3 hourly 4 times daily for 3 days.
Neuralgia of face	:	**Causticum 200** 1 drop with half spoon cold water once daily morning for 10 days.

Aviod Cosmetics.

Right sided facial neuralgia	: **Chelidonium 200** 1 drop with half spoon cold water 6 hourly 2 times daily for 5 days.
Left sided facial neuralgia	: **Thuja 200** 1 drop with half spoon cold water 6 hourly 2 times daily for 5 days.
Spasm in any part of the face	: **Cuprum Met. 200** 1 drop with half spoon cold water half hourly 4 times a day.
Vermilion redness of lips	: **Sulphur 30** 2 drops with half spoon cold water 2 hourly 4 times daily for 2 days.
Bright redness with swelling of lips	: **Graphites 30** 2 drops with half spoon cold water 2 hourly 4 times a day.

Smoking is injurious to health.

EYE

The eye is a delicate organ which encroaches the first position among other sensasory organs. The eye is a mirror of life. Without vision, life is miserable.

The Eye is located in a nature protected cavity of the skull bones. The lids and the eye lashes aid in protecting the visual organ anteriorly. The muscles in the orbit of eye is called the **Orbicularis Oculi**. The mechanism of this muscle initiate closing of eye lids. The other muscle at the back of orbit is called **Levator Palpebrae Superioris** which initiate opening of the upper eye lids. An epithelial membrane in front of the eye protects the pathogenic bacteria that may enter from outside. The natural flow of tears wash away all foreign objects from the eye.

The eye ball consists of two types of muscles called **Intrinsic** and **Extrinsic**. The Intrinsic muscles are of two circular structures to govern the performances of the Pupil, which is the central opening of the pigmented part called **Iris**. The extrinsic muscles are attached to the bones of eye orbit and extended upto the outer most white layer (Sclera) of the eye ball.

Extend your helping hands to a blind person.

The eye is a delicate organ because of its function and mechanism. The eye ball has three different layers as mentioned below :

I) Sclera : Outer most white layer with firm connective tissues as a protective wall to combat foreign objects.

II) Choroid : This second layer contains dark brown pigment and a net work of connective tissues. This layer prevents incoming light or rays.

III) Retina : This innermost coat contains 10 layers of nerve cells and the receptors called **Rods** and **Cones** for identifying colours. The Rods are sensitive to white and black i.e. bright and dark. The Cones are sensitive to red, green, and blue. The Optic Nerve carries visual impulses of the Rods and Cones to the visual interpretation area of Occiputal lobe. The Opthalmic Nerve carries impulses of touch, pain and encroachment by foreign bodies.

The refracting mechanism of the eye is hidden in the structures as narrated below :

I) Cornea : It is the window of the eye. It is a forward continuation of the transparent outer coat. It is the prime pathway of light rays. It bulges forward slightly.

II) Aqueous Humor : It is watery fluid in front of the crystalline lens. It maintains the forward curve of the Cornea. It has two bulging surfaces for biconvex purpose.

An ounce of prevention is worth a pound of Cure.

Eye

III) Crystalline: It is a jelly-like substance located in a circular structure. The mechanism of elasticity of this lens regulates the near or distant vision.

IV) Vitreous : It is also a jelly-like substance located body behind the lens and maintains the spherical shape of the eyeball and aid refraction.

The Iris, pupil and ciliary body also plays a vital role relating to visual activities. The circular muscle fibres of the Iris rugulate the entrance of light to the eye. It protect strong light by reducing the size of the central opening (pupil). But when the light is less, the muscles contract and initiate enlargement of the pupil.

Similarly, the pupil reduce its size when viewing a nearby object. But when viewing a distant object, the pupil enlarges.

The ciliary body maintains the refracting ability of the lens.

The Conjunctiva covers the anterior part of the Sclera and protect the eyeball from drying. The watery secretion from the **Lacrimal Gland** keep the conjuctival sac moist. The Lacrimal gland is located in the upper part of the orbit. Tears also flow from the Lacrimal gland.

INTERPRETATION OF VISION :

Light enters the eye through its pathway called **Cornea** and reaches first to the **Crystalline Lens** and then to the **Vitreous Body**. Due to refraction at the bulging surfaces, an image is formed on the Retina. The receptors (Rods & Cones) carries the impulses to the visual interpratation area of brain through **Optic Nerve**. Thus 'Seeing' is possible.

Neglegency carry risk.

Diseases :

Mal-formation or irregularities in muscular, nervous and lens may cause conginatal blindness. Total colour blindness may cause due to defective Cones.

Partial colour blindness may cause to the persons those who lack of one type of Cone. Colour blindness is an inherited condition and occur almost in males. Vitamin/ Mineral defficiency, Mechanical injury, Welding sparks, smoke from Cigarettes/ Bidis, close watch of T.V./Video, use of unadjusted spects, Eclipse burn, leakage inside the eye, damage of Optic Nerve, Retinal haemorrhage, old age, may lead to the following diseases.

1. Myopia (Shortsightedness)
2. Hypermetropia (Long-sightedness)
3. Presbyopia (Blurred vision)
4. Photophobia (Aversion to light)
5. Cataract (Clouding of Lens due to Metabolic or Age related conditions)
6. Retinitis (Haemorrhage from the retinal blood vessels.
7. Macular Oedema (Accumulation of fluid due to rupture or leakage from Retinal blood vessels)
8. Glaucoma (Damage of Optic Nerve due to irregular pressure of Aqueous Humor fluid)

In such conditions, it is suggested to consult Opthalmologist without delay.

Eye Care :

Any one may suffer from eye troubles. Hence a special care should be taken as preventive measure. Self

Eye

medication may lead to several complications. Viewing green objects is beneficial for eye sight. It could be observed that the eye complications are comparatively less among the Tea garden labourers, farmers which may be possible due to their nature of job with green leaves that too within a natural green surroundings.

Diabetic patients must ensure periodical eye check-up and control diet within a limit of 1800 K. cal per day. Diabetes may lead to various eye complications.

Habit of taking sufficient green vegetables and salads daily, viewing green objects, bare-footed walk on grass lawn are essential for maintaining normal eye sight. Moreover, Vitamin A containing food items like Butter, Carrots, Sweet Potatoes, Spinach, Yellow vegetables ,fish liver oil, Orange, Mango and Tomato should be taken regularly. Tomato may be ranked first as a preventive against night blindness, short sightedness, weakness of Optic nerve.

'**Carotenoids**' are very much essential to prevent Cataract. The availability sources of Carotenoids are dark green leafy vegetables and red fruits.

The following common ailments of eye may be treated under Homoeopathic system of medicines.

Inflamation of eyes	: **Arnica Mont. 30** 2 drops with half spoon cold water 3 hourly 4 times daily for 5 days.
Painful soreness of eyeballs	: **Eupatorium 30** 2 drops with 1 spoonful cold water 3 hourly 3 times daily for 3 days.

See and let see.

Pupils insensible to light	: **Merc. Cor.30** 2 drops with half spoon cold water once daily for 10 days.
Pupils dialated	: **Helleborus Niger 200** 1 drop with 1 spoonful cold water 1 hourly 4 times daily for 3 days.
Tired feeling in eyes	: **Ruta Grav. 200** 1 drop with half spoon cold water 2 hourly 3 times a day.
Severe burning & soreness of eye.	: **Merc. Cor. 30** 2 drops with half spoon cold water 1 hourly 4 times daily for 2 days.
Swelling of eye lids	: **Apis Mel.30** 2 drops with half spoon cold water half hourly 4 times daily for 2 days.
Pain just above eyes	: **Chinonanthus Virginica Q** 3 drops with 2 spoonful cold water 4 hourly 3 times daily for 2 days.
Pain over the eyes	: **Bryonia Alb. 200** 1 drop with half spoon cold water 3 hourly 3 times daily for 2 days.
Flow of tears from eyes	: **Euphrasia 200** 1 drop with half spoon cold water 3 hourly 4 times daily for 2 days.
Bruised pain in eyes while moving.	: **Cuprum Met. 200** 1 drop with half spoon cold water 3 hourly 4 times a day.

Eye is the pearl gifted by God.

Eye

Mechanical injury to eye ball	: **Symphytum 30** 3 drops with 1 spoon cold water 4 times at 15 mnts. interval.
Dim Vision	: **Ruta Grav. 200** 1 drop with half spoon cold water daily morning for 15 days.
Eyes red due to cold exposure	: **Belladonna 30** 2 drops with half spoon cold water 4 times daily at 15 mnts. interval.
Conjunctivitis with lacrimination	: **Argentium Nitrate 200** 1 drop with half spoon cold water half hourly 4 times daily for 3 days.
Paralysis of eye lids	: **Causticum 200** 2 drops with half spoon cold water once at morning daily for 10 days.
Rainbow colour flickering before eyes.	: **Phosphorus 30** 2 drops with half spoon cold water 3 hourly 4 times daily for 3 days.
Styes on eye lids	: **Staphisagria 200** 1 drop with half spoon cold water 3 hourly 4 times daily for 2 days.
Soft Cataract	: **Cineraria Maritima Succus.** 2 drops in each eye to be applied twice daily at morning and evening for 1 month.

Strong medicines have strong reactions.

Hard Cataract	: **Conium 3x** 3 drops with 2 spoon cold water 3 hourly 4 times daily for 1 month.
Double Vision	: **Gelsimium 200** 1 drop with half spoon cold water 3 hourly 4 times daily for 3 days.
Eyes feel hot	: **Ruta Grave.200** 1 drop with half spoon cold water 3 hourly 4 times daily for 2 days.

■■

EAR

The particular shape, curves of the human ear and its inner organs like **Eardrum, Stirrup, Hair Cells** and other natural mechanism maintains the hearing system.

The ear canal amplifies speech sound frequencies. The ear-drum attached with **'Stirrup'**, formed with a chain of three smallest bones on a tiny Snail shaped organ which contains necessary fluids. There are several thousands of hair-cells on the membrane which covered the fluid. The sound carried to the fluid first and subsequently to the hair-cells which communicate the speech to the brain after necessary filtration (frequency limit). Then the anterior temporal lobe of the brain governs memory through audio, visual and physio-motor system.

Without pleasure of sound and speech, a life is miserable. A new born baby also enjoy the rythm of sound and speech. Gradually, imitation and natural trial starts with speaking of broken words from infant stage. Such expressions can be possible when audio system is normal. Because, one can't react without proper hearing. A child with conginatal hearing deformaties may not be vocal and such condition obviously causes intellectual

---

Noise pollution leads to deafness.

Conginatal deformaties with Low-set or Marfans (prominent ears), heriditary, mechanical injury, deep ear abscess, cystic growth inside ear canal, typhoid, small-pox, infiltration of any foreign body, accumulation of wax. lack of concentration are the prime causes behind temporary or permanent deafness.

Apart from those factors, the hearing system may be affected due to sound pollution.

The sound is measured in **Decibel** (dB). A normal human voice may be measured within a range of 30-40 dB. As the inner ear cells are able to tolerate sound upto 85 dB normally, any kind of hearing difficulties may develop when the sound exposure exceeds 100 dB. A sudden sound exposure like thundering, bomb explosion, blasts are more harmful in comparison to continuous sound exposure from the roaring industrial machineries. aeroplane, micro-phone, vehicular traffic and sharply blown horn etc. In case of any complicacy, it is wise to consult ENT specialist for necessary check-up and treatment.

It may not be out of place to mention here that the habit or speaking with loud voice may lessen hearing sensibility. Better try to be a good listener with regular practice of excercise as given below :

* Concentrate on speeches while hearing.
* Make response only after clear hearing.
* React on speeches but not on speakers.
* Do not talk irrelevent.
* Tune voice while speaking to others.
* Better talk less.

Tune voice while speaking.

Ear

However, the following medicines are found much effective for treatment of some common ailments relating to Ear.

Earache due to wax inside	: **Mullein Oil Q** 4 drops to be applied in each ear twice daily. **Chamomilla 200** 1 drop with half spoon cold water half hourly 3 times a day.
Earache due to cold exposure	: **Aconite Nap. 30** 2 drops with 1 spoon cold water half hourly 4 times a day.
Earache affecting head	: **Belladonna 200** 1 drop with half spoon cold water 3 times a day at 15 mnts. interval.
Mild and long lasting earache	: **Pulsatilla 200** 1 drop with half spoon cold water 3 hourly 3 times daily for 2 days.
Earache with one cheek red and hot	: **Chamomilla 30** 1 drop with half spoon cold water 1 hourly 3 times daily for 3 days.
Earache with swelling of the ear canal	: **Aconite Nap. 30** 2 drops with half spoon cold water half hourly 4 times daily for 2 days.

Keep surroundings free from noise pollutions.

Humming sound inside ear	: **Graphites 30** 1 drop with half spoon cold water half hourly 4 times daily for 2 days.
Roaring sound inside ear	: **Sulphur 30** 2 drops with one spoon cold water 1 hourly 3 times a day for 2 days.
Buzzing sound inside ear	: **Dulcamara 30** 2 drops with half spoon cold water 1 hourly 3 times daily for 2 days.
Bleeding from ear	: **China 30** 2 drops with half spoon cold water half hourly 4 times a day.
Pus secretion from ear	: **Pulsatilla 200** 1 drop with half spoon cold water 6 hourly 2 times daily for 3 days.
Sudden deafness	: **Phosphoric Acid 30** 2 drops with half spoon cold water 1 hourly 3 times daily for 3 days.
Erruption inside or around ear	: **Graphites 200** 2 drops with a spoonful cold water 2 times daily at morning and evening for 2 days.
Catarrhal inflamattion of middle ear.	: **Merc. Cor. 30** 2 drops with half spoon cold water 1 hourly 3 times daily for 4 days.

■■

Today's negligency : tomorrow's repentation

NOSE

The Nose is a vital organ because of its duel performances like breathing and sensasory organ for smell.

The Nasal structure consists of a pair of bones (Conchae) and a blunt blade shaped bone (Vomer). There are two seperate spaces within the nasal cavities, located between the upper part of the Mouth and Cranium. The spaces are separated by a thin partition known as Nasal Septum.

Due to the particular shape of conchae, air makes its entrance initially to the nasal cavity through Nostrils and then to the Lungs through the Pharynx and Trachea. Similarly, all gaseous waste products are also expelled through nostrils. The nose is a vital organ for maintaining respiratory system by inhaling and exhaling of air through nostrils and the process is known as **Breathing**.

The Vascular membranes of the nasal cavities contains many blood vesels and thin hairs which protects entrance of dust particles, pathogens and foreign bodies during inhalation of air. The nose performs primary filtration of air before communicating to Lungs.

The Receptors for Smell in the **Olfactory Epithelium** are located in the extreme upper interior part of the nose. The receptors carries the impulses to the Olfactory centre in the Brain through the **cranial nerve** for interpretation of smell. The sense of taste is also closely related to smell interpretation.

The **Maxillary Sinus** communicate with the nasal cavities. The Nasolacrimal duct inside the nasal cavities produce tears and keep the Conjuctivital Sac moist.

The nasal cavity is very much sensitive. The sudden exposure to sun/cold, vehicular fumes, smoke from burning rubber products, coal, tar, artificial sneezing habit, addiction to smoke or sniff, inhalation of strong perfumes, adenoids, pollypus may cause obstruction to Smell interpretation and also lead to various complicacies like Epistaxis (bleeding from nostrils), running nose (coryza), catarrhal discharge, nasal voice, continuous sneezing etc.

The following Homoeopathic Medicines are found effective for treatment of some nasal problems as mentioned below :

Running Nose : **Camphor 30**
2 drops with half spoon cold water 3 times a day at 15 mnts interval.

Frequent sneezing due to dust allergy : **Sulphur 30**
2 drops with half spoon cold water half hourly 3 times a day.

Infection inside Nose : **Merc. Cor 30**
3 drops with a spoonful cold water 4 hourly 3 times daily for 3 days.

Nose bleeding (Epistaxis) : **Carbo Veg. 30**
2 drops with half spoon cold water half hourly 4 times a day.

Natural food is vital food

Nose

Nasal pollypus	: **Calcarea Carb. 30** 3 drops with a spoonful cold water once at morning daily for 15 days.
Pain in nasal bone	: **Drossera 200** 1 drop directly on tongue once at morning daily for 7 days.
Sinus congestion	: **Kali-Bi-Chrom. 200** 2 drops with a spoonful cold water 3 hourly 3 times daily for 3 days.
Coryza	: **Allium Cepa 30** 3 drops with a spoonful cold water 4 times daily at 15 mnts. interval.
Smell of old catarrah	: **Sulphur 200** 1 drop with half spoon cold water once at morning daily for 10 days.

■■

LIPS

The **Lips** plays multifarious role including opening of mouth, control of voice, facial expression, smile and facial beauty.

The ring-shaped muscular system of **Lips** is called **Orbicularis Oris**. This muscle encircles mouth and its antagonists regulates closing and opening of the lips, expression of a smile.

The following Homoeopathic Medicines are found effective for the treatment of Lips :

Ulcerated patches inside lips
: **Carb. Ac. 30**
2 drops at a time with 1 spoon cold water 3 hourly 3 times daily for 4 days.

Burning around lips
: **Anacardium 30**
2 drops at a time with half spoon cold water 1 hourly 4 times a day.

Crack lips
: **Nit. Acid 30**
3 drops at a time with 1 spoon cold water 3 hourly 3 times daily for 3 days.

Avoid cosmetics.

Lips

Crack upper lip	: **Baryta Carb. 30** 2 drops at a time with 1 spoon cold water 3 hourly 3 times daily for 3 days.
Crack in corners	: **Natrum Mur.30** 2 drops with 1 spoon cold water 3 hourly 3 times daily for 3 days.
Vesicles on lower lip with burning	: **Sepia 30** 2 drops with 1 spoon cold water 3 hourly 3 times daily for 2 days.
Sticky discharge from lips	: **Graphites 30** 2 drops with 1 spoon cold water 3 hourly 4 times daily for 5 days.
Swelling of upper lip	: **Apis Mel. 30** 2 drops with half spoon cold water 1 hourly 4 times daily for 2 days.
Swelling of lower lip	: **Kali-bi-Chrom.30** 2 drops with half spoon cold water 1 hourly 3 times daily for 2 days.
Ulcers in upper lip	: **Causticum 30** 2 drops with 1 spoon cold water 4 hourly 3 times daily for 2 days.
Ulcers in lower lip	: **Sepia 30** 3 drops with a spoonful cold water 4 hourly 3 times daily for 5 days.

Nature is the best healer.

Lips red and easily bleeding	: **Kreosotum 30** 3 drops with a spoonful cold water once daily for 7 days.
Pimples on lips	: **Mur. Acid 30** 2 drops with half spoon cold water once at morning daily for 10 days.
Lips black and swollen	: **Merc Cor. 30** 3 drops with a spoonful cold water 3 hourly 3 times daily for 5 days.
Partial paralysis of lower lip	: **Glonoin 30** 2 drops with half spoon cold water 4 hourly 3 times daily for 10 days.

■■

MOUTH

The **Mouth** is the oral cavity with various accessory organs like tongue, teeth, parotid glands (near the ear), submaxillary glands (near the lower jaw), sublingual glands (under the tongue) and palate inside. The oral cavity is covered by a large muscle called - Buccinator .

Because of its shape and flexibility, this is also known as **Trumpeter's muscle** which helps in whistling , blowing and accomplishment of speech and breathing casually.

Food is necessary for nourishment and the mouth with flatten cheek is having natural mechanism to receive food and process for supply to the digestive system through the **Alimentary Canal.**

The accessory organs start functioning as soon as the mouth receive any food. The teeth carry out chewing (mastication) while the tongue rotate the food and perform swallowing (deglutition). The glands - **Parotid, Submaxillary** and **Sublingual** produces necessary saliva for processing food and swallowing.

For the treatment of some common ailments related to mouth, the following Homoeopathic medicines are found effective :

Torn wounds inside the mouth	: **Calendula 30** 2 drops with half spoon cold water 3 hourly 3 times daily for 5 days.
Bleeding from any part of mouth	: **Acid Nitrate 200** 2 drops with half spoon cold water 4 times a day at 15 mnts. intervals.
Ulcers inside the mouth	: **Acid Nitrate 30** 2 drops with half spoon cold water 3 hourly 3 times daily for 5 days.
Dryness of mouth	: **Pulsatilla 200** 1 drop with half spoon cold water 1 hourly 4 times a day.
Lock Jaw	: **Hypericum 30** 4 drops with half spoon cold water 4 times at 10 mnts. interval.
Blisters inside the cheek	: **Arsenic Alb. 30** 3 drops with a spoonful cold water 3 hourly 3 times daily for 2 days.
Foul smell from mouth	: **Helleborus Niger 200** 1 drop with half spoon cold water once daily morning for 10 days.

■■

Smoking is injurious to throat

TOOTH

The necessity of **teeth** is better known to all from childhood to old age. A variety of liquid and solid food are the natural nutrient which supply Carbohydrate, Protein, Fat, Vitamins, Minerals and Water for maintaining body system. All children need food for growing well and adults need food for physical fitness to live. But consumption of solid food may not be possible without the help of teeth.

The tooth is nothing but a living tissue known as **Dentin**. It is coated with a hardest substance known as **Enamel**. The nerve (Pulp) inside **Dentin,** is closely connected with Gum for maintaining firmness and carryout supply of necessary minerals, Vitamins for dental system.

Due to biological demand for solid food, a phase-wise dentition starts from the age between 6 to 8 months during infancy. Dentition ceases after erruption of total 32 teeth with equal break-up of 16 teeth in upper and lower jaw. Each set comprised of 2 Central Incisors, 2 Lateral Incisors, 2 Canines, 4 First Molars, 4 Second Molars, 2 Third Molars (Wisdom Teeth) which are of different size and shape corresponding to upper and lower jaw. Out of 32, the deciduous teeth (Temporary teeth commonly known as Milk Teeth) are 20 in number. A table showing the normal dentition period is as follows :

Teeth	Normal Dentition Time	
	Temporary	*Permanent*
Central Incisors	6 to 8 months	6 to 8 years
Lateral Incisors	7 to 11 months	7 to 9 years
Canines	1 year 4 months to 1 year 8 months	9 to 12 years
First Premolars } Second Premolars }	—	10 to 13 years
First Molars	10 months to 1 year 4 months	6 to 7 years
Second Molars	1 year 8 months to 2 years 6 months	12 to 13 years
Third Molars (Wisdom Teeth)	—	17 to 25 years

Regarding the get-up of teeth, **Incisors** are flat in shape with partial sharp edges, **Canines** with pointed edges and comparatively large shaped **Molars** with flat edges.

Due to improper cleaning of teeth, mounting of food particles is obvious and which in the long run may form a sticky white film (Plaque) on the tooth surface. Accumulation of food particles also produce bacteria which are prone to damage the hardest enamel coating of teeth and cause cavity. Such condition is enough for causing tooth decay, sensitivity to hot or cold contacts, affect on gum and surrounding bones, formation of pus, bleeding, stomach trouble, severe toothache and other sufferings

Cleanliness is Heavenliness.

Tooth

including difficulties in consumption of necessary food and even cancer.

Apart from irregularities, depletion of Minerals (Calcuim, Phosphorus, Fluorine) and Vitamin-C (Fruits, Lemon, Oranges, Gooseberies, Guava), Genetic influence, pollution of water and environment may attribute to loose teeth, decay and scurvy etc.

A dental research in Spain recently, confirmed that leaded petrol fumes from vehicular traffic may cause air pollution to a maximum extent. Lead from vehicular fumes may go directly into the teeth or through blood stream. Such air pollution may damage the coating of enamel which protects the tooth.

It is wise to realise the utility of teeth well in advance and prevent decay. A proper attention to the following oral hygiene rituals are absolutely necessary for maintenance of teeth.

* Use of quality tooth paste and comfortable soft tooth brush.
* Regular Gum massage with index finger.
* Brushing of teeth thrice daily at morning, mid- day and before going to bed at night.
* Sugar or Carbohydrate rich food may cause damage to tooth enamel.
* Flossing of interdental area with tepid water after taking milk, sweet dishes, chocholate, fruits etc.
* Never traumetize teeth or gum by pins, match sticks or tooth picks.
* Contact of wooden pencil lead with teeth may cause harm to a maximum extent.

Natural food is vital food.

* Never indulge in eating together in a same dish or glass.
* Tobacco, Pan Masalas, Smoking may promote discolouration of teeth.
* Opening of bottle caps with teeth may cause damage to tooth as well as enamel.
* Cutting of nails with teeth is also prejudicial.
* In case of any problem with loose or painful tooth, it is wise to consult a Dentist and extract the disturbing teeth.
* Fibreous food like sugar cane, orange, apple, mango etc. also serves cleaning of teeth.
* A balanced diet including the following Vitamins and Minerals is absolutely necessary for protection of teeth.

Vitamin : C (Lemon, oranges, Gooseberies, guava etc.)

Minerals : Calcium (Milk, Butter, Green leafy vegetables).

Phosphorus (Cereals, Pulses, Milk etc.)

Fluorine (water, Milk, Fruit juice).

The following medicines are found effective for the treatment of some dental diseases in acute stage.

Delayed dentition : **Calcarea Carb. 30**
2 drops with half spoon cold water 3 hourly 3 times daily for 10 days.

Smile is free : distribute freely.

Tooth

Teething convulsion	: **Belladonna 30** 2 drops with half spoon cold water 1 hourly 3 times daily for 3 days.
Faulty teeth	: **Calcarea Carb. 30** 2 drops with half spoon cold water once daily morning for 1 month.
Jerking toothache	: **Coffea Cruda 30** 2 drops with half spoon cold water 4 times at 10 mnts. interval daily till recovery.
Constant Toothache	: **Plantago M. Q** For local application once or twice daily.
Toothache due to carries	: **Kreosotum 30** 2 drops with half spoon cold water 3 times at 15 mnts. interval daily.
Severe Toothache	: **Apis Mel. 30** 2 drops with half spoon cold water 3 times at 15 mnts. interval daily.
Enamel defficiency	: **Calcarea Carb. 30** 2 drops with half spoon cold water once daily morning for 30 days.
Gum Swelling	: **Merc. Sol. 30** 2 drops with half spoon cold water 2 hourly 3 times daily for 3 days.

Good health is the noblest gift of God

Loose Teeth	: **Acid Nitricum 30** 2 drops with half spoon cold water 3 hourly 2 times daily for 15 days.
Falling of lower jaw	: **Helleborus Niger 30** 2 drops with half spoon cold water half hourly 3 times daily for 5 days.
Gum Bleeding	: **Merc. Cor. 30** 2 drops with a spoonful cold water half hourly 4 times daily for 2 days.

■■

TONGUE

The **Tongue** is very important among other sensasory organs like Eye, Ear, Nose and Skin. It has two types of muscles called **Extrinsic** and **Intrinsic**. The extrinsic muscle cover the outer part and the intrinsic muscles are within the tongue. The tongue has much flexibility due to two fold muscular system and a particular shape as necessary for its easy movement while speaking, chewing and swallowing.

The tongue muscles are connected with Taste buds (receptor),**Facial nerve, Glossopharyngeal nerve, Hypoglossal nerve** and the **Salivary glands** like **Submaxillary, Sublingual** and **Lacrimal.**

The tongue can perfectly detect the taste which are essentially of four kinds- Sweet, Sour Salty, and Bitter. The taste receptors (taste buds) which are located along the edges of very small depressed areas (fissures) of the tongue carry taste impulses to the brain through the connective nerves for detection of taste. The taste buds in the anterior two thirds of the tongue can detect the taste as given below :

1. Sweet tastes are detected at the tip of the tongue.
2. Sour tastes are detected at the sides of the tongue.

Maintain oral Hygiene.

3. Salty tastes are detected at the front part of the tongue.

4. Bitter tastes are detected at the back part of the tongue.

The Facial Nerve with sensasory fibres are involved with the detection of taste. This nerve also contains secretory fibres to the smaller **Salivary** glands like Submaxillary, Sublingual and Lacrimal.

The **Glossopharyngeal nerve** contains general sensasory fibres from the back of the tongue and the pharynx. But the sensasory fibres of this nerve are located at the posterior third of the tongue for taste detection. The motor nerve fibres keep control over the swallowing muscles in the **Pharynx** and the **Hypoglosal** nerve is for controlling the muscles of the tongue and carrying impulses. The largest salivary gland, (Parotid), regulate the secretory fibres of the tongue.

The tongue may loose its sensitivity due to regular consumption of liquor, hot tea, coffee or milk, chewing of tobacco, pan masala, smoking or uncleaned condition, fungal infection, bite form loose teeth or broken teeth, apthae etc. Nervousness causes stammering. Better maintain a clean and mild voice while speaking to babies. In case of any irregularities or erruptive condition of tongue, it would be wise to consult a specialist for immediate medical treatment.

The Tongue infection by **Fungus Candida** albieans is very much common among the bottle-fed babies due to sucking of rubber made nipples or mother's infected nipple. Such fungal infection may spread its affect to the gastrointestinal and respiratory tract which is of great risk.

Smoking is injurious to health

Tongue

In such cases, child specialist must be consulted immediately.

The following Homoeopathic medicines have proven to be very effective for cure of some common diseases of tongue as given below :

White Fungal coating on tongue	: **Antimonium Crud. 200** 1 drop with half spoon cold water 3 hourly 4 times daily for 2 days.
Tongue coated with white thick mucus.	: **Merc. Cor. 30** 3 drops with 1 spoonful cold water 3 hourly 4 times daily for 2 days.
Painful vesicles on tongue	: **Veretrum Alb.30** 2 drops with half spoon cold water 2 hourly 3 times daily for 3 days.
Crack tongue	: **Borax 30** 2 drops with 1 spoonful cold water 4 hourly 3 times daily for 3 days.
Tongue white with red tip and edge.	: **Sulphur 30** 2 drops with half spoon cold water 2 hourly 3 times daily for 2 days.
Constant taste of salt	: **Iodium 30** 2 drops with 1 spoonful cold water 3 hourly 3 times daily for 2 days.
Metallic taste	: **Merc. Cor. 30** 3 drops with 1 spoonful cold water 3 hourly 3 times a day.

Eat green vegetables

Sweetish taste	: **Cumprum Met. 30** 2 drops with 1 spoonful cold water 4 hourly 3 times daily for 2 days.
Constant salivation	: **Merc. Cor. 30** 2 drops with 1 spoonful cold water 2 hourly 4 times daily for 3 days.
Ulcer on tongue	: **Acid Nitricum 30** 2 drops with 1 spoonful cold water 2 hourly 3 times daily for 3 days.
Any mechanical injury on tongue	: **Arnica Mont. 30** 3 drops with 1 spoonful cold water half hourly 4 times daily till recovery.
Paralysis of tongue	: **Causticum 200** 1 drop with half spoon cold water once daily morning for 7 days.
Stammering	: **Stramonium 200** 1 drop with half spoon cold water once daily morning for 10 days.
Apthae of tongue	: **Borax 200** 1 drop with half spoon cold water 3 hourly 3 times daily for 3 days.

■■

Breath fresh air

THROAT

The **Throat** is a complicated but important part of the body. It has a complex muscular system known as **Sternomastoids**. This muscular system initiate flexibility and easy movement of the head. A strong muscle known a **Trapezius** muscle (extended from shoulder) is also located at the back of neck to support the head. It may be mentioned here that spasm of the muscles or severe injury causes stiffness of the neck. In such cases, the movement of the head may not be possible. This condition is known as **Torticollis** (wry neck).

There are two arteries known as **Carotid** located in the both sides of the **Adams Apple**. The Carotid in the right side supplies blood to right side of head and neck. The other Carotid located at the left side of the neck supplies blood to the left side of the head and neck.

The extreme upper part of the **Vertibral Column** is in the neck. This part is called **Cervical Vertebrae**. There are 7 numbers of vertebrae in the neck.

The inner portion of the throat is more complex as it carry out multifarious activities including breathing, swallowing and speech (voice).

Smoking is injurious to health.

Pharynx, the beginning portion of the **Alimentary Canal** is often referred to as the **Throat** which starts from the ending part of the tongue. The upper part of the Pharynx is located behind the nasal cavity and known as **Nasopharynx**. The middle part behind the mouth is called **Oropharynx** and the lowest part is called **Laryngeal Pharynx**. It is located in a juncture point. The front portion makes way for air into the Larynx and the back portion makes way for food to the **Oesophagus**. Just below the **Laryngeal Pharynx**, the Larynx (Voice box), **oesophagus** and **Trachea** are located one after another. The trachea conduct air supply between larynx and lungs. The larynx is located between pharynx and trachea. Commonly the larynx is larger in male in comparison to female. For which, female voice is thin (low). It has a frame work of **Cartilage** known as **Adam's Apple**. It is commonly seen in the front part of the neck of some male having thin and long shaped neck.

The space between two vocal cords is called **Glottis**. A leaf shaped trapdoor like fleshy lid closes this opening during swallowing food and helps diversion to the oesophagus. Simultaneously, this trapdoor rises while breathing and allow air inside. This trapdoor is called **Epiglottis**.

At the beginning of the throat, a nipple shaped mass hangs from the central part of the Soft Palate. It is called Uvula. It plays vital role to conduct swallowing and proper movement of food and also control speech (voice).

Besides, there are different masses of **Lymphoid** tissue in the throat for filtration of tissue fluid. These are known as **Tonsils**. The oval shaped Tonsils are located at the each side of the **Soft palate** and the junction between the opening of the **Oesopharynx** and

---

Natural food is vital food

Pharynx. These are known as **Paletine Tonsils**. Another Tonsil is located on the back wall of the upper Pharynx. It is known as Pharyngeal Tonsil. The another type of small Tonsils known as **Lingual Tonsils** which are located at the back of the tongue. Tonsils play an important role to defend the body against allergic diseases and prevent the entry of possible micro organism through the throat and protect the respiratory tract and lungs from infections and fight against the diseases.

Thyroid Gland is also located in the throat. This is the largest of the **Endocrine glands** (the glands without ducts and supply its secretions to various body tissues through blood and lymph). It has two oval shaped parts known as **Lateral Lobes** and located one on either sides of Voice box. The **Thyroid Gland** produce **Calcitonin Hormone** which is essential for Calcium metabolism in the body system. Moreover the Thyroid gland produces **Thyroxine** and **Triodothyronine** hormone which regulates mental and physical activities and growth of the body. The Parathyroid glands are located behind the Thyroid. These are 4 in number. These glands produces **Parathormone** hormone which increases Calcium level in blood. It regulates exchange of Calcium between blood and bones.

As the throat is a gateway of air and food, any kind of infection in the throat is obvious for creating various difficulties. The guard like Tonsils are very much sensitive. These are often infected due to cold or hot exposures, inhalation of dust, environmental pollution, damp surroundings, improper ventilation, intake of contaminated water, addiction to liquor or Smoke, chewing of tobacco. The ailments like enlargement, septic condition, presence of pseudomembrane on the tonsils, hoarseness of voice, Diptheria, difficult swallowing, unpleasant taste in the mouth, reccurrent coughs, hiccough, throat pain extending up to ears, Cancer and increased susceptibility to other infections including Bronchitis, Bronchial Asthma and Sinusitis.

The **Iodine** defficiency causes irregularities in Thyroid functioning. Malfunctioning of Thyroid may lead to the ailments like general debility, inflamation of the neck, Goitre, Stiff neck, retarded growth. Similarly, the irregularities in parathyroid glands may lead to some complicacies like contractions of face and hand muscles, tumours of the parathyroid, easy fracture of bones, formation of stones in the Kidney.

The following Minerals/Vitamins are necessary for maintaining healthy condition of mouth and throat.

Minerals :
1. Iodine (Iodized Salt, Sea fish).
2. Phosphorus (Cereals, Pulses, Milk, Banana).
3. Copper/Cobalt (Cereals, Pulses, vegetables, Meat).
4. Sulphur (Cereals, Pulses).

Vitamins :
1. Vitamin -C (Fresh fruits, Lemon, Orange, Gooseberries, Guava & Banana).
2. Vitamin - D (Fish, Liver, Oil, Milk and exposure to Sun).
3. Vitamin - B2 (Green leafy vegetables, Peas).

In case of any irregularities in the throat, it is wise to consult ENT specialist for necessary Checkup and treatment without delay.

Strong medicines have strong reactions.

Throat

The following Homoeopathic Medicines are found very much effective for the treatment of throat.

Sore throat	: **Arnica Montana 30** 2 drops at a time 2 hourly 4 times a day with half spoon cold water.
Malignant Sore throat	: **Muriatic Acid 30** 3 drops with half spoon cold water 3 hourly 4 times daily for 4 days.
Throat ulcers	: **Acid Nitricum 30** 3 drops with half spoon cold water 4 hourly 4 times daily for 7 days.
Throat Abcess	: **Merc. Cor. 30** 3 drops with half spoon cold water 3 hourly 4 times daily for 7 days.
Throat congestion	: **Belladona 30** 2 drops with half spoon cold water 3 hourly 4 times a day.
Oedematus swelling of throat	: **Apis Mel. 30** 3 drops with half spoon cold water 1 hourly 3 times daily for 3 days.
Suppurating sore throat	: **Merc. Cor. 30** 2 drops with half spoon cold water 4 hourly 3 times daily for 4 days.
Sensation as if a plug in throat.	: **Hepar Sulphur 200** 2 drops with 1 spoon cold water 3 hourly 4 times a day.

Health is wealth; preserve it

Pricking sensation in throat.	: **Argentinum Nitricum 30** 3 drops with half spoon cold water 1 hourly 3 times a day.
Sticky discharge from throat	: **Kali-Bi-Chrom 200** 1 drop with half spoon cold water 3 hourly 4 times daily for 5 days.
Inflamation of Uvula	: **Kali-Bi-Chrom 30** 3 drops with 1 spoon cold water 3 hourly 4 times daily for 3 days.
Ulcers in Uvula	: **Iodium 30** 3 drops with 1 spoon cold water 3 hourly 3 times daily for 5 days.
Salivation	: **Merc. Cor. 30** 3 drops with 1 spoon cold water 4 hourly 3 times daily for 5 days.
Carotid congestion	: **Belladonna 30** 3 drops with 1 spoon cold water 1 hourly 3 times daily for 2 days.
Cough with vomiting due to throat irritation	: **Ipecacuanha 30** 3 drops with 1 spoon cold water 1 hourly 4 times a day or two.
Inflamation of tonsils	: **Phytolacca B. 30** 2 drops with half spoon cold water 3 hourly 3 times daily for 7 days

Drink sufficient water.

Throat

Suppurating tonsils	: **Baryta Carb. 30** 3 drops with 1 spoon cold water 3 hourly 3 times daily for 7 days.
White spots in tonsils	: **Merc.Iod. Flavum 30** 2 drops with half spoon cold water once at morning daily for 10 days.
Inflamed Thyroid	: **Iodium 30** 3 drops with 1 spoon cold water 3 hourly 4 times daily for 10 days.
Difficult swallowing of food	: **Baptisia 200** 2 drops with 1 spoon cold water 3 hourly 3 times daily for 3 days.
Pharyngitis	: **Hepar Sulph 30** 2 drops with 1 spoon cold water 3 hourly 3 times daily for 5 days.
Diptheria	: **Phytollacca B.30** 3 drops with 1 spoon cold water 3 hourly 3 times daily for 10 days.
Mild Diptheria	: **Baptisia 200** 2 drops with 1 spoon cold water once daily morning for 7 days.
Malignant Diptheria	: **Amon Carb. 30** 2 drops with 1 spoon cold water 3 hourly 4 times daily for 10 days.

Food is energy

Hiccough (Hiccup)	: **Ipecacuanha 30** 3 drops with half spoon cold water half hourly 3 times a day.
Laryngitis	: **Argentinum Nitricum 200** 2 drops with 1 spoon cold water 4 hourly 3 times daily for 5 days.
Broken voice	: **Causticum 200** 2 drops with half spoon cold water 1 hourly 3 times daily for 3 days.
Mumps	: **Belladonna 30** 3 drops with 1 spoon cold water 2 hourly 3 times daily for 5 days.
Mumps with earache	: **Phytolacca B. 30** 2 drops with 1 spoon of cold water half hourly 4 times daily for 3 days.
Ulcers in Oesophagus	: **Iodium 30** 3 drops with 1 spoon of cold water 3 hourly 4 times daily for 7 days.

■■

Cleanliness is heavenliness

HAND

In human body, the extremities are divided into two sections i.e. upper and lower extremities. The upper extremities include the shoulders, upper arms, forearms, wrists, hands and fingers. The lower extremities include the limbs of leg. In the upper extremity, there are 32 bones as described below :

The arm (shoulder to elbow) bone is known as **Humerus** which hangs from the shoulder blade known as **Scapula** (a part of shoulder **girdle**).

There are two bones in the forearm (elbow to wrist) known as **Ulna** (lies on the medial) and **Radius** (lies on the lateral i.e. inner side parallel to the thumb).

The wrist contains eight small **Carpal** bones Viz. **Hamate, Pisiform, Triquetral, Lunate, Lesser Multangular Greater Multangular, Capital, Navicular.**

The body of the hand (palm) is a framework of five metacarpal bones.

There are 14 finger bones (2 in thumb and 3 for each finger) called phalanges. The phalanges attached to Metacarpal bones are called **Proximal** and others known as **Distal phalanges.**

Low diet causes defficiency diseases

The Trapezius muscles located in the shoulder and neck also cover a part of the upper arm. These muscles helps in raising of shoulder.

The **Latissimus Dorsi** muscles helps extension and bringing down the arm. Without such action of the muscles, swimming may not be possible.

The **Pectoralis Major** muscles in axilla (armpit) is an extended muscle from the chest. This muscle helps in pulling the hands across the chest.

The **Serratus Anterior** muscles below the axilla (armpit) aids in raising the arm. This also helps in pushing or pressing.

Just below the shoulder, the **Deltoid** muscle in the upper arm helps in raising the hand to the horizontal position. The **Biceps** muscle flexes fore arm and the Triceps muscle extends the fore arm.

The muscles in the anterior part of the elbow is known as Olecranon.

The Flexor Carpi and Extensor Carpi muscles conduct many movements of the hand. The fexor Digitorum and Extensor Digitorum group muscles located in the forearm, regulate movement of the fingers.

The Deltoid muscles in the upper arm is often used for administering intermuscular injections.

The human body contains nearly 300 pairs of Skeletal muscles. The pair of muscles are of two types i.e. **Prime Mover** and **Antagonist**. Muscular movement is initiated by the Prime mover. When an opposite movement is to be made, the Antagonist takes over. All muscular movements are carried out by the co-ordinated movements of the Prime Mover and Antagonist.

Keep diet balance

Hand

For maintenance of blood circulatory system in the hands, there is a network of Principal Arteries and Principal Veins as mentioned below :

Arteries :
1. Subclavian
2. Axillary
3. Brachial
4. Radial
5. Ulnar
6. Volar Arch
7. Volar Metacarpals
8. Volar Digitals

Veins :
1. Cephalic
2. Basilie
3. Median Cubital
4. Brachial (same as the corresponding arteries
5. Axillary -(same as the corresponding arteries)
6. Subclavian -(same as the corresponding arteries)

For Blood pressure monitoring, the **Sphygmomanometer** cuff is wrapped in the upper arm to obstruct the blood flow of the Brachial Artery.

For counting the Pulse rate, a mild pressure with the fingers on the Radial Artery is done near the wrist.

Intervenus Medication (injections) are administered through the largest group of Veins viz. **Cephalic, Basilic** and **Median Cubital**.

The hands plays prime role in human life with two fold activities - destructive and constructive. The plans,

---

Natural food is vital food.

idea originate from the brain but can't be achieved or implemented without co-ordination of hands. All inventions, creative or destructive, are the contribution of hands. However, a sound hand boosts up the ability of earning bread and butter. Depletion of minerals/vitamins, prolonged illness and particularly lack of morale/ confidence may develop diseases in any part of the body including hands.

To keep the systems of hands active, regular exercise, swimming are most essential. Balanced diet including the following minerals/vitamins are absolutely necessary to get rid of some common diseases like rheumatism, gout, numbness of muscle, stiffness, jerking of hands, trembling of muscles.

Minerals:	Potassium:	(Fruits)
	Calcium:	(Milk, Milk products Eggs, Greenleaf, vegetables, Banana).
	Phosphorus:	(Cereals, Pulses, Milk, Banana).
	Magnesium:	(Green leaves, Cereals).
Vitamins:	B12 :	(Meat, Fish).
	D :	(Fish, Liver, Oil, Milk, exposure to sunlight).
	Ascorbic Acid:	(Cirtrus fruits, Green veg-etables)
	Pantothenic Acid.	(Liver, Eggs, Yeast).

The following Homoeopathic medicines are found effective for treatment of some common ailments related to hands.

Swimming is the best exercise.

Hand

Pain in joints	: **Ruta G. 200** 2 drops with 1 spoon cold water 4 hourly 3 times daily for 2 days.
Pain in shoulder joints	: **Chelidonium 30x** 2 drops with 1 spoon cold water twice daily at morning and evening for 5 days.
Muscular contraction	: **Causticum 200** 1 drop with half spoon cold water 3 hourly 4 times daily for 7 days.
Rheumatic pain in shoulder.	: **Sanguinaria Can. 200** 2 drops 1 spoon of cold water once daily morning for 10 days.
Twitching of muscles	: **Cuprum Met. 200** 2 drops with a spoonful cold water half hourly 3 times daily for 2 days.
Numbness of limb	: **Causticum 200** 1 drop with half spoon cold water 4 hourly 3 times daily for 7 days.
Partial paralysis of hands.	: **Glonoin 30** 3 drops with 1 spoonful cold water 3 hourly 3 times daily for 3 days.
Spasm in fingers	: **Cuprum Met 200** 2 drops with 1 spoonful cold water half hourly 4 times a day.

Low diet causes deficiency diseases.

Crack palm	: **Alumina 200** 2 drops with 1 spoonful cold water once at morning daily for 10 days.
Painful wrist	: **Ruta G. 200** 2 drops with 1 spoonful cold water 3 hourly 3 times daily for 5 days.
Jerking of hands	: **Gelsemium 200** 2 drops with a spoonful cold water half hourly 3 times daily for 5 days.
Coldness of hands.	: **Cuprum Met 200** 2 drops with half spoon cold water once at morning daily for 7 days.
Swelling of muscles	: **Apis Mel. 30** 3 drops with 1 spoonful, cold water half hourly 4 times daily for 2 days.
Septic fingers	: **Hypericum Q** To be applied on the affected fingers daily 3 times.
Pain in palm	: **Apis Mel. 30** 3 drops with 1 spoonful cold water 3 hourly 3 times daily for 3 days.
Burning palm	: **Cantharis 200** 2 drops with 1 spoonful cold water 3 hourly 3 times daily for 2 days.

Prevention is better than cure

Hand

Itching palm	: **Petrolium 200** 2 drops with 1 spoonful cold water half hourly 3 times daily for 3 days.
Convulsion of fingers.	: **Cuprum Met. 200** 2 drops with half spoon cold water 3 hourly 3 times daily for 3 days.
Crack nails	: **Hypericum Q** For local application 3 times daily on nails for 2 months. **Antimonium Crud. 200.** 1 drop with 1 spoon cold water once daily morning for 5 weeks.

■■

Avoid alcoholic drinks

CHEST

The **Thoracic Cavity** in the chest is the prime part of the body which contains the **Heart,** the **Lungs** and **Aorta**. This cavity is located just above the abdominal cavity. Both the cavities are seperated by the **Diaphragm,** a muscular partition. The Thoracic cavity is covered by a cage shaped 24 ribs (12 pair) which are attached to the Vertebral column posteriorly and Sternum anteriorly. The first 7 pair of ribs from the upper part are connected with the Sternum by means of costal cartilages. the 8th, 9th and 10th pairs are united to each of the cartilage. The rest 11th and 12th pairs are floating. This frame work of bones called- **Thorax** which guard the vital organs as mentioned above. There are three sacs in the Thoracic cavity.: two **Pleural Sacs** of Lungs in the left and right side and a **Pericardial** Sac in the Heart.

The Diaphragm is a muscle that contracts and elevate the ribs with the help of muscles- external intercostals between ribs. This process helps enlargement of the Thoracic cavity which is absolutely necessary for respiration.

The main functions of the organs in the Thoracic cavity are as follows :

Breath fresh air.

Chest

1. **Heart** : This vital organ is slightly bigger than a fist. It is located in the Pericardial Sac in the centre between the Lungs. The heart is a hollow organ with three tissue layers : **Endocardium** (Smooth layer), **Myocardium** (thickest layer) and **Pericardium** (forms the outermost layer).

    The human heart is a double pump and its two sides are completely seperated from each other by a thick partition called Septum but they work together. On either side, there are two chambers called **Receiving chamber** and **Pumping chamber**. The receiving chamber carries out function with **Right Atrium** and **Left Atrium**. The Right Atrium receives the blood returning form the body tissues which is low in Oxygen and carried to the veins. The left Atrium receives blood high in Oxygen as it returns from the Lungs.

    The pumping chamber carries out its function with **Right Ventricle** and **Left Ventricle**. The right Ventricle pumps the venous blood received from Right Atrium and sends the blood to the lungs. The Right Ventricle pumps oxygenated blood to all parts of the body through the Arteries. The following 4 valves are located at the entrance and exit of each Ventricle.

    I. **Tricuspid Valve** is known as the **Right Atrioventricular** Valve. It has three openings and closing flaps. When this valve is open, blood flows from the Right Atrium to Right Ventricle and enter into the Pulmonary Artery.

    II. **Pulmonary Semilunar Valve** is located between the Right Ventricle and the Pulmonary Artery which leads to the Lungs. The valve prevents the back flow of blood.

Frequent exposure to X-Ray is injurious to health.

III. **Left Atrioventicular Valve (Mitral Valve)** has two thick flaps (cusps) which conduct transfer of blood from Left Atrium to Left Ventricle which supply blood into the Aorta. The flaps prevent back flow of blood.

IV. **Aortic Semilunar Valve** is located between the Left Ventricle and Aorta. It prevents the back flow of blood from the Aorta to the Ventricle.

Blood Pressure : The heart pumps blood into the blood vessel (Arteries) which supply blood all over the body. When the heart contracts to pump, blood rushes into the blood vessels. This is called **Systolic Blood Pressure** (Upper). But when the heart relaxes, the pressure is called **Diastolic Blood Pressure** (Lower). The blood Pressure is measured in Milimeters of Mercury (mm hg). The device **'Sphygmomanometer'** is used for monitoring blood pressure. This device is available in the following three types :

- Mercury
- Aneroid (Dial type)
- Electronic (Digital)

Normal range of blood pressure :

Systolic Pressure : 100 to 140 mm hg. at any age.

Diastolic Pressure : 60 to 90 mm hg. at any age.

Grades of Blood Pressure :

Normal upper limit   : 140/90 mm hg.
Mild Hypertension   : 150/95 to 160/100 mm hg.
Moderate Hypertension: 160/100 to 180/110 mm hg.
Severe Hypertension   : 180/110 to 220/120 mm hg.

Good health is the noblest gift of God.

Caution : In case of severe Hypertension, it is wise to monitor Blood Pressure at least 3 times at different intervals. If Blood pressure is persistently high every time, then only it can be considered a case of high blood pressure. Because, the blood pressure may go up temporarily due to excitement., anxiety, panic, mental stress, diabetes, over weight and high Cholestoral level in blood. The blood pressure comes back to normal rate when the temporary stress is over. Moreover, if the instrument is very old or the cuff around the arm is very loose or tight, it can give a false high reading. So the Blood pressure should be checked properly in lying position.

Special Care should be taken to ensure :

* Regular check up
* Weight reduction
* Smoking/intake of alcohol should be avoided.
* Checking of Cholestoral level in the blood and to ascertain HDL and LDL cholestoral ratio.
* Daily walk for 45 mnts.
* Yogic exercise like **Shabasana** with **Pranayama** regularly.
* Adequate rest.
* Consumption of seasonal fruits in plenty.
* To take minimum quantity of salt daily. Total curtailment of salt may reduce Sodium level of blood which causes fatigue, nervous debility and muscu lar cramps.

In case of Hypertension (High B.P.), a low Sodium diet is suggested as follows:

Break Fast : 1 cup of Tea/Coffee with required sugar and milk

---

Smoking is injurious to health.

Mid morning	:	1 apple
		2 biscuits
		2 chapattis
Lunch	:	2 chapattis
		1 cup dal
		1 cup rice
		1 bowl cooked green leafy vegetables.
		1 bowl salad
Dinner	:	1 cup Tomato soup (add little milk)
		2 toasted vegetable sandwiches
		1 bowl rice
		1 cup curd
Bed time	:	1 glass of hot milk without sugar.

2. **Lungs** : It is the organ of respiration which serve to conduct breathing i.e. rythmic inhalation (drawing of air into the Lungs) and exhalation (expulsion of air from the Lungs). Drawing of air is the active phase and expulsion of air is the passive phase of breathing.

There are two Lungs side by side in the **Thoracic Cavity**. Each lung is well sealed in a membranous sac called the **Pleura**. Both the pleurae are associated with each lung. The muscular **Pharynx** (see Throat chapter) serves as a passage for air into the respiratory tract and the **Trachea** (Wind pipe) conduct air between Larynx and the Lungs. At a particular space just behind the heart, the trachea divides into two branches called- **Bronchi**. The right Bronchi is larger in diameter than left Bronchi. As soon as the bronchus

---

Ill health invites more inllness.

enters the Lung, it subdivides as the branches of a tree for thorough distribution of air into the lungs.

The inhaled air contains a mixture of Oxygen, Nitrogen, Carbon dioxide and other gases. But only Oxygen is necessary for survival.

Respiration has two aspects : external and internal. External respiration takes place in the spaces which include the Nasal cavities, the Pharynx, the Larynx, the Trachea and finally the Lungs where Oxygen from surface air enters the blood and Carbon dioxide is removed from the blood. Internal respiration conduct gas exchanges between the blood and the body cells through the capillaries of the **Alveoli** (cluster of air sacs). Oxygen leaves the blood and enters the cells while Carbon dioxide leaves the cells and enters the blood. The Pulmonary circuit brings the blood to and from the Lungs. The following are the respiratory control centres :

- Medulla (a part of the brain)
- Pons (a part of the brain)
- Phrenic Nerve to Diaphgram.
- Chemoreceptors (Carotid and Aortic bodies).

3. **Aorta** : It is the largest and continuous artery (blood vessel) with the following four divisions :

   I. **Ascending Aorta** - located near the heart and inside the **Pericardial Sac.**

   II. **Aotic Arch** - curves from the right to left and extends backward.

   III. **Thoracic Aorta** - lies behind the heart and in front of the Vertebral Column.

   IV. **Abdominal Aorta** - covers the abdominal cavity.

Prevention is better than cure.

Exposure to cold, depletion of Vitamins/Minerals, unhealthy atmosphere and inadequate ventilation, environmental pollution, addiction to alcohol/smoke, over eating, obesity, diabetes, stress, anxiety, fear etc. may cause various diseases in the Thoracic cavity.

The following Homoeopathic medicines may be kept handy.

Weak feeling in chest	: **Acid Phos 30** 2 drops with 1 spoonful cold water 3 hourly 3 times a day.
Breathing trouble	: **Apis Mel 6x** 3 drops with 1 spoonful cold water half hourly 4 times for 3 days.
Shortness of breathing	: **Calcarea Carb.30** 2 drops with half spoon cold water 3 times at 15 mnts interval.
Weak sensation about the chest and Heart.	: **Iodium 30** 3 drops with 1spoonful cold water 3 hourly 2 times daily for 3 days.
Chest pain	: **Bryonia Alb. 200** 2 drops with a spoonful cold water half hourly 3 times a day.
Chest pain during deep breathe	: **Calcarea Carb. 30** 3 drops with 1 spoonful cold water once at morning daily for 7 days.

Ensure proper ventillation.

Chest

Palpitation of heart	: **Iodium 30** 3 drops with 1 spoonful cold water half hourly 2 times daily for 5 days.
Great anxiety and palpitation of Heart.	: **Calcarea Carb. 6** 4 drops with a spoonful cold water 3 times at 15 mnts. interval.
Cardiac distress at night	: **Arnica Mont. 200** 2 drops with 1 spoonful cold water 3 times at 15 mnts. interval.
Difficult breathing while lying	: **Amonia Carb. 30** 2 drops with a spoonful cold water once at morning daily for 7 days.
Shortness of breath while going upstairs	: **Iodium 30** 3 drops with 1 spoonful cold water once at morning daily for 10 days.
Sudden chest pain	: **Acid Nitricum 30** 3 drops with 1 spoonful cold water 3 times at 10 mnts. interval.
Cramps in chest muscles	: **Cuprum Met. 200** 2 drops with 1 spoonful cold water 3 hourly 3 times daily for 3 days.
Inflamation of lungs	: **Belladonna 3 x** 4 drops with 1 spoonful cold water 3 hourly 3 times daily for 7 days.

Ensure balanced diet

Inflamation of pleura	: **Aconite Nap. 30** 3 drops with 1 spoonful cold water 2 hourly 3 times daily for 5 days.
Air hunger	: **Carbo Veg. 200** 2 drops with half spoon cold water 4 times at 10 mnts. in-terval a day in acute stage. In chronic case-2 drops with 1 spoon cold water once at morning daily for15 days.
Bleeding from lungs	: **Acid Nitricum 30** 3 drops with 1 spoon cold water 1 hourly 3 times daily for 7 days.
Bleeding from lungs due to pthisis	: **Acalypha Indica Q** 5 drops with half cup cold water 3 hourly 2 times daily for 10 days.
Difficult breathing due to rattling of mucus in chest.	: **Antim Tart. 30** 3 drops with 1 spoon cold water half hourly 3 times a day.
Blood with sputum	: **Iodium 30.** 3 drops with 1 spoon cold water 3 hourly 3 times daily for 7 days.
Cough at night only	: **Petrolium 30** 3 drops with 1 spoon cold water 2 hourly 2 times daily evening for 3 days.

Prevention is better than cure

Chest

Suffocative cough	: **Cuprum Met 200** 2 drops with 1 spoon cold water half hourly 3 times a day.
Whooping cough	: **Drossera 30** 3 drops with 1 spoon cold water 3 hourly 3 times daily for 7 days.
Thick cough with foul smell	: **Kreosotum 200** 2 drops with 1 spoon cold water once at morning daily for 10 days.
Cough with vomiting	: **Ipecac 30** 3 drops with 1 spoon cold water half hourly 4 times daily for 3 days.
Thick/dry cough with chest pain	: **Bryonia 200** 2 drops with 1 spoon cold water 3 hourly 2 times daily for 10 days.
Cough without expectoration	: **Hepar Sulph. 200** 2 drops with a spoon cold water 3 hourly 3 times daily for 3 days.
Face bluish due to suffocative cough.	: **Lobelia 30** 3 drops with 1 spoon cold water half hourly 2 times daily for 3 days.
Rapid respiration due to severe cough.	: **Ipecac 30** 3 drops with half spoon cold water 3 times at 10 mnts. interval a day.

Health is wealth - preserve it

Hard cough with sound of a driven saw.	: **Spongia Tosta 30** 3 drops with 1 spoon cold water 2 hourly 3 times daily for 3 days.
Asthma	: **Blatta Orientalies Q** 6 drops with half cup cold water 6 hourly two times daily for 15 days.

■■

ABDOMEN

The abdominal cavity is located below the **Thoracic** cavity. **Diaphragm** is a partition between both the cavities. The abdominal cavity is covered by **Peritoneum**. The abodomen is also covered by a three-tier muscular system called-(1) external oblique (out side), (2) Internal oblique (middle) and (3) transversus abdominis (innermost). The abdominal muscles protect the sensitive organs inside and due to flexible shape, the muscles aid the process of respiration and other functions. The abdominal cavity is divided into the following 9 regions:

1. **Right hypochondriac region** : located in the right upper part just below the right chest.

2. **Left hypochondriac region** : located in the left upper part just below the left chest.

3. **Epigastric region** : located in the centre between right and left hypochondriac regions.

4. **Right lumber region** : located just below the right hypochondriac region.
5. **Left lumber region** : located just below the left hypochondriac region.
6. **Umbilical region** : located between the right and left lumber region.

Over eating is harmful.

7. **Right Iliac region** : located in the right lower abdomen i.e.below the right lumber region.
8. **Left Iliac region** : located in the left lower abdomen i.e.below the left lumber region.
9. **Hypogastric region** : located between the right and left iliac region.

The following are the chief organs and their functions inside the abdominal cavity.

1. **Stomach** : It is an enlarged part of the Alimentary Canal. This part is located just below the Diaphragm. A ring like muscle called Sphincter at the upper part of the stomach regulates entrance of food and another Sphincter at the lower part contricts the passage for retention of food for process and act as the exit of stomach. The Sphincter in upper part is called **'Esophageal Sphincter'** and the lower part sphincter is called **'Pyloric Sphincter'**. The stomach is flexible due to its muscular shape and system. After retention of food, the glands in the stomach wall start secretion of digestive enzymes (Pepsin, Gastric juice etc) which has two main components : (1) **Hydrochloric Acid** (2) **Enzymes**. The hydrochloric acid in the stomach juice kills bacteria and other disease producing agents if any enters with food. Apart from this, the hydrochloric acid activates stomach enzymes which are essential for liquifying of food and partial digestion. The longest **Cranial Nerve**-(Vagus) supplies digestive juices to the glands inside the abdominal cavity. The digestion is a process for conversion of food into the basic materials like carbohydrates, fats, proteins, mineral salts, vitamins and water for supply to the body cells. The distribution system is known as 'absorption'. The entire system of food processing continue through the **Alimentary Canal** which is the longest canal starting from the mouth and

---

Keep Diet Balance.

Abdomen

extending to the rectum. It is composed of several parts : Pharynx, Oesophagus, Stomach, Small intestine and Large intestine. The entire system of food processing continue through the Alimentary Canal.

2. **Liver** : The largest gland 'Liver' is located in the right hypochondriac region (right upper abdomen) under the dome of the diaphragm. It has several functions including storage of Glycogen (Glucose) for necessary supply into the bloodstream when blood sugar level comes down, formation of Albumin, Fibrinogen and Blood Plasma, proteins, modification of fats, synthesis of urea, manufacture of Bilirubin, Bile, removal of poisonous properties, manufacture of Heparin that prevents clotting of blood and supply digestive juices through a duct of Duodenum.

The Liver has four lobes. The right lobe is larger in shape than that of left one and two other lesser lobes. The Portal Vein and the Hepatic Artery deliver nearly 1-1/2 quarts of blood to the Liver every minute.

When the food is digested and absorbed from the Small Intestine into the blood stream, and transported to the Liver by the portal circulatory system, the Liver process the nutrients for supply into the general circulation.

3. **Gall Bladder** : It is a muscular sac on the outer side of the Liver and serves for bile storage. The Liver produced bile flows into the Gall Bladder through the Liver ducts. When the processed food with gastric juice enters through Duodenum, the Gall Bladder contracts and for which bile rushes into a duct leading to the Duodenum.

4. **Pancreas** : The pancreas is a ductless (endocrine) gland. Due to absence of ducts, the endocrine glands are dependent upon the blood and the lymp to carry the hormones to various body tissues by way of the capillar-

Low Diet causes deficiency diseases.

ies of the glandular tissue. But the pancreas contains both Exocrine and Endocrine gland tissue. There are small groups of cells called '**Islets;** (Islets of Langerhans) which function independently with necessary secretion of **Insulin** to transport Glucose into cells and produces Glucagon which stimulates the Liver to release Glucose.

The secretion of enzymes- Amylase, Trypsin and Lipase from the Pancreas acts on starches, proteins and fats of the digested food in the small intestine.

5. **Spleen** : It is a gland like organ located in the left upper part (left hypochondriac region) of the abdominal cavity which serves as reservoir for blood. It is involved with various functions : breakdown of old Red Blood Cells, formation of Red Blood Cells, destruction of bacteria, formation of Lymphocytes and Monocytes.

6. **Small Intestine** : The Small Intestine is the longest part (20 feet approx) of the Alimentary Canal and located just below the Stomach in the following three divisions : First 10- 12 inches below the stomach is called Duodenum, second major part is called- Jejunum and the remaining part is called Ileum which joins the large Intestine through a Valve. The diameter of the Small Intestine is smaller than Large Intestine.

The Small Intestine secretes its own juice (Lactase, Maltase, Sucrace) and breaks down fats so that Pancreatic juice Lipase can digest them (absorption), the means by which the digested food (energy) reaches the bloodstream and finally transported to the Liver through **Portal circulatory System**

7. **Duodenum** : It is about 10-12 inches long upper part of the Small Intestine. In the Duodenum is an opening into which lead two ducts called Pancreatic Duct (carry Pancreatic juice) and common Bile Duct (carry bile from liver and gall bladder).

Natural food is vital food.

Abdomen

8. **Common Bile Duct** : The single duct leading to the opening of Duodenum carry out supply of bile for digestion of fats from the Liver as well as Gall Bladder.

9. **Large Intestine** : The Large Intestine carry out excretion of waste materials after digestion and absorption process in Stomach and Small Intestine. It is known as Colon which comprises of four divisions : (1) **Ascending Colon** (2) **Transverse Colon** (3) **Descending Colon** and (4) **Sigmoid Colon**. It is larger than small Intestine in diameter. At the beginning, there is a small pouch called the **Caecum** which is the junction of the small and large Intestines. This juncture point is located in the right lower Iliac region of the abdomen. A Small blind tube hanging below the Caecum is called the **Vermiform Appendix**. The Ascending Colon extends upward form the Caecum and bends to the left side of the abdomen forming the **Transverse Colon**. Finally the Colon bends downward on the left side of the abdomen into the pelvis. This subdivision is called the Descending Colon. The lower part of the Descending Colon is called the **Sigmoid Colon** which empties into the **Rectum**.

The two Kidneys lie against the muscles of the back in the upper abdomen.

The lower part of the abdominal cavity is called - pelvic Cavity in which are located the Urinary Bladder, Prostate Gland (in male persons) and other internal parts of the male and female reproductive system. The rectum is also in the **Pelvic Cavity**.

The following are the Homoeopathic remedies for treatment of most common abdominal disorders.

Gastralgia : **Arsenic Alb. 30**
3 drops with 1 spoon cold water 3 hourly 3 times daily for 3 days.

Vegetarian food is easily digestable.

Abdomen

Pain abdomen	: **Nux Vomica 3x** 4 drops with 1 spoon cold water half hourly 4 times daily for 2 days.
Gastric distrubances	: **China 30** 3 drops with 1 spoon cold water 1 hourly 3 times a day.
Gastric disturbances in upper abdomen	: **Carbo Veg.200** 2 drops 1 spoon cold water 3 hourly 2 times at morning daily for 5 days.
Gastric disturbances in lower abdomen	: **Lycopodium 200** 2 drops with a spoonful cold water 2 hourly 2 times daily evening for 3 days.
Burning pain in stomach	: **Merc. Cor. 30** 3 drops with 1 spoon cold water half hourly 4 times daily till recovery.
Pricking pain in abdomen	: **Acid Nitricum 30** 3 drops with half spoon cold water half hourly 4 times only.
Shooting pain in upper abdomen	: **Ignatia 200** 2 drops with 1 spoon cold water 1 hourly 3 times a day.
Violent cutting pain in abdomen	: **Cuprum Met. 30** 3 drops with 1 spoon cold water half hourly 4 times only.
Bloated abdomen	: **Iodium 30** 3 drops with half spoon cold water 1 hourly 3 times only.

Food is energy.

Abdomen

Gastric disturbances	: **Pulsatilla 30** 2 drops with half spoon cold water half hourly 3 times a day.
Stiching pain in right upper abdomen.	: **Berberis Vul. 200** 2 drops with 1 spoon cold half hourly 4 times daily till recovery.
Pain in left upper abdomen	: **Ceanthus 200** 1 drop with half spoon cold water 2 hourly 3 times daily.
Pain abdomen due to Gall Bladder Stone.	: **Chelidonium 6** 4 drops with 1 spoon cold water half hourly 4 times a day.
Pain abdomen due to over eating	: **Bryonia Alb.200** 2 drops with half spoon cold water half hourly 3 times a day.
Pain in right lower abdomen due to early appendicitis	: **Belladonna 200** 2 drops with 1 spoon cold water 3 hourly 3 times daily for 4 days.
Appendix region tender & painful	: **Ignatia 200** 2 drops with 1 spoon cold water 3 hourly 2 times daily for 7 days.
Distention with Vomiting	: **Helleborus Niger 30** 3 drops with 1 spoon cold water half hourly 3 times a day.
Chronic Diarrhoea	: **Calcarea Carb. 30** 3 drop with 1 spoon cold water 3 hourly 3 times daily for 10 days.

Strong medicines have stong reactions.

Abdomen

Involuntary Diarrhoea	: **Apis Mel.30** 3 drops with 1 spoon cold water half hourly 4 times daily for 3 days.
Watery stool with cutting pain in abdomen.	: **Cuprum Met. 30** 3 drops with half spoon cold water 4 times at 15 mnts. interval.
Green Diarrhoea	: **Argent Nitrate 30** 3 drops with 1 spoon cold water 1 hourly 3 times daily for 3 days.
Diarrhoea after taking food or drinks	: **Arsenic Alb.30** 4 drops with 1 spoon cold water half hourly 4 times daily for 3 days.
Diarrhoea with vomiting:	**Veretrum Alb. 30** 3 drops with 1 spoon cold water 4 times at 10 mnts. interval.
Diarrhoea alternated with constipation.	: **Iodium 30** 3 drops with 1 spoon cold water once at morning daily for 10 days.
Vomiting and severe pain in stomach	: **Bryonia Alb. 30.** 2 drops with half spoon cold water 4 times at 10 mnts. interval.
Vomiting with nausea	: **Nux Vomica 30** 3 drops with 1 spoon cold water 4 times at 10 mnts. interval.

Cleanliness is Heavenliness.

Abdomen

Vomiting after drinks	: **Arsenic Alb.30** 2 drops with half spoon cold water half hourly 4 times a day.
Voilent vomiting relieved by drinking cold water	: **Cuprum Met.30** 3 drops with 1 spoon cold water half hourly 4 times a day.
Simple Dysentery	: **Merc. Sol.30** 3 drops with 1 spoon cold water half hourly 4 times daily for 3 days.
Blood Dysentery	: **Merc. Cor. 30** 4 drops with half spoon cold water 4 times at 10 mnts. interval daily.
Dysentery with blood & mucus	: **Iodium 30** 3 drops with a spoonful cold water 4 times at 10 mnts. interval daily.
Dysentery with pain abdomen	: **Colocynth 30** 2 drops with half spoon cold water 4 times at 15 mnts. interval.
Dysentery with burning Anus	: **Capsicum 200** 2 drops with 1 spoon cold water 2 hourly 3 times daily for 3 days.
Constipation	: **Bryonia Alb. 30** 3 drops with 1 spoon cold water once at morning daily for 15 days.

Donate blood and save a life.

Constipated stool like hard small balls.	: **Opium 30** 4 drops with 1 spoon cold water once at morning daily for 15 days.
Severe constipation	: **Plumbum 12** 3 drops with 1 spoon cold water once at morning daily for 15 days.
Hungry feeling at pit of stomach	: **Sulphur 30** 3 drops with 1 spoon cold water half hourly 4 times a day.
Heart burn after food	: **Calcarea Carb. 30** In acute case : 3 drops with 1 spoon cold water half hourly 3 times only. In chronic Case : 2 drops with 1 spoon cold water once at morning daily for 15 days.
Severe burning in stomach	: **Carbo Veg. 200** 2 drops with 1 spoon cold water 3 hourly 2 times daily for 5 days.
Burning intestine	: **Iris 30** 2 drops with 1 spoon cold water 1 hourly 3 times daily for 3 days.
Irregular liver function and loss of appetite.	: **Carica Papaya Q** 15-20 drops with half cup of cold water twice daily for 7 days.
Enlarged Liver	: **Kalmegh Q** 10 drops with half cup of cold water twice daily before principal meals for 15 days.

All covet, all lost.

Abdomen

Jaundice	: **Chelidonium 200** 2 drops with 1 spoon cold water 3 hourly 3 times daily for 10 days.
Gargling sound in stomach at morning hours.	: **Sulphur 30** 3 drops with 1 spoon cold water 3 hourly 3 times daily for 4 days
Gargling sound in stomach at evening hours	: **Lycopodium 200** 2 drops with 1 spoon cold water once at evening daily for 5 days.
Worms	: **Cina 3x** 4 drops with 1 spoon cold water 3 hourly 3 times daily for 7 days.
Pain abdomen due to Worms	: **Atista Indica Q** 5 drops with half cup of cold water 2 hourly 3 times a day.
Tape Worm	: **Calcarea Carb 6** 3 drops with half spoon cold water once at morning daily for 30 days.
Purgative	: **Aegle Folia Q** 8 drops with half cup of luke-warm water once at morning.

■■

Now is the time to compare vegetarian and non- Vegetarian Animals

URINARY SYSTEM

The **Kidney** is the vital organ which regulates retention of necessary volume of water as body fluid and excretion of excess water as urine.

Before explaining the Urinary System, it is necessary to make focus on the location, structure and functions of the kidney.

A pair of **Kidney** in the body system is located in a well protected space in the upper abdomen under the dome of the diaphragm. The space is known as **Retroperitoneal space**. The normal size of each Kidney is 4 inches (10 cm) long, 2 inches (5cm) wide and 1 inch (2.5cm) thick. The artery, veins and the ureters are connected with the Kidneys. Each Kidney is covered by a membranous capsule called **Adipose capsule**. The outer part is known as **Renal Cortex** and innermost part is **Renal Medulla**. The Medulla is connected with several structures called **Pyramids**. The outer part called Renal Pelvis is connected with the Ureters. The prime part of the Kidney is called **Nephron**, a coiled tube microscopic in size, regulate entire renal functions. Two small glands called **Adrenal glands** are located at the top of the Kidneys.

Drink sufficient water.

Urinary system

The function of the Kidneys include the following :

1. Maintenance of Water Balance In The Body :

The Cells in the body depends on the constancy of fluid. To keep the cells active, the body maintains storage level of water from 50% to 75%. Out of which, a major volume of water is necessary for the cells. This is called **Intracellular Water**. The remaining volume is necessary for storage outside the cells and within blood. The volume outside the cells is known as **Extracellular Water** and the volume runs with blood is **Plasma**. The fall of water level causes **'dehydration'** i.e. imbalance in Electrolytes.

Hypothalamus, which is located just above the **Pituitary Gland** maintain the Thirst mechanism. As and when the water level comes down, the Hypothalamus sends messages demanding water. The tongue and throat turns dry and the individual drinks water for recovery of fluid.

For biological process, the substances dissolve in body water turns into Electrolytes, a composition of the following salts :

- Sodium : necessary of stimulation of nerves.
- Potassium : necessary to convert Carbohydrate as energy.
- Calcium : necessary for bone formation, blood clotting and maintenance of muscular activities.
- Phosphate : essential for cells and metabolism of Carbohydrate.
- Chloride : produce Hydrochloric Acid for gastric juice.

2. Regulating Acid-Base Balance :
A certain proportion of acids and bases are necessary for body function.

Avoid use of public Toilet.

The body gets acids or bases from some foods and cell metabolism. The Kidney regulates the acid-base balance as per need of the body.

3. **Production of Hormones** : The Adrenal glands produce hormones called **Adrenaline** which aids the muscular contraction, blood pressure balance, conversion of Glycogen of the Liver into sugar during emergency and normal heart beat.

The **Adrenal Cortex** produces **Cortisol** which is necessary of maintaining a reserve stock of Carbohydrate in the body by conversion of **Amino Acids** into Sugar. The reserve stock of Carbohydrate protects the body during stress.

The **Aldosterone** hormone from the Adrenal Cortex aids in regulating body electrolytes. The Kidney also produces some other hormones for various purposes. The secretion of **Renin** from the kidney acts on the vascular system and stimulating bone marrow.

4. **Regulating Urinary System** : Both the kidneys regulate the urinary system through its components - a pair of **Ureter**, a single **Urinary Bladder** and single **Urethra**. The ureters carry the waste products discharged from the kidneys and pass on to the urinary bladder. Commonly the Ureters are 10-12 inches (25 cm - 32 cm)long which varies with the height of the individual. The urinary bladder is a reservoir for urine and located below the **Peritoneum** behind the pubic joint. The length of the bladder is 2 inches (5 cm) but it is flexible upto 5 inches (12.5 cm) when carry the collected volume of urine (nearly 470 ml). The urethra is a narrow tube extends from the urinary bladder to out side through the genital. The main function of the urethra is to drain out urine from the bladder. Such excretion is called urination (micturition). The size and

---

Prevention is better then Cure.

Urinary system

function of the urethra differs in men and women. In male persons, about 8 inches (20 cm) long urethra passes through the **Prostate** gland and ends as the outlet of **Glans penis**. The **Spermatic Cord** is connected with the male urethra in a juncture point of prostate gland. There are two ejaculatory ducts at the juncture point of the urethra. Just below, there is another gland known as **Couper's gland** in the male urethra. The male urethra serves duel purpose i.e. drainage of urine from the bladder and carrying seminal fluid. The duct regulates the flow.

The female urethra is about 3.75 cm long and located behind the pubic joint and extend upto the front wall of the vagina. The female urethra is the outlet of urine only.

The normal colour of urine is pale yellow. The normal specific gravity of urine is 1.010. If there is any disorder in the urinary system and irregularities in kidney functioning, the specific gravity varies upto 1.040. Commonly urine carry the following substances :

Urea, Uric acid, Creatine, Sodium Chloride, Sulphates, Phosphate and Yellow pigment.

Diabetes Mellitus, Rheumatism, Gout, High Blood pressure (Hypertension), irregularities in the Endocrine gland system, mental stress, alcoholic drinks, intake of less water, consumption of protein food beyond limit are the prime causes behind the kidney diseases.

The following Homoeopathic medicines are recommended for immediate treatment of common ailments as mentioned below.

Scanty Urine : **Helleborous Niger 200**
2 drops with 1 spoon cold water 1 hourly 3 times daily for 3 days.

Strong medicines have strong reactions.

Urinary system

Suppressed Urine	: **Merc. Cor. 30** 4 drops with 1 spoon cold water 2 hourly 4 times daily for 3 days.
Urine passed in drops	: **Apis Mel. 30** 3 drops with 1 spoon cold water 4 hourly 3 times daily for 5 days.
Frequent effort but passed a few drops.	: **Eupatorinum 30** 2 drops with 1 spoon cold water half hourly 4 times daily for 3 days.
Painful urination	: **Apis Mel. 30** 3 drops with 1 spoon cold water half hourly 4 times daily for 2 days.
Dreads to urinate due to hot and burning urine.	: **Borax 30** 3 drops with 1 spoon cold water 4 times at 10 mnts. interval.
Burning in Urethra	: **Merc. Cor. 30** 3 drops with 1 spoon cold water 4 times at 15 mnts. interval daily.
Involuntary Urination (Enuresis).	: **Pulsatilla 30** 2 drops with half spoon of cold water 3 hourly 3 times daily for 5 days.
Frequent urination at night.	: **Argent Met. 6x** 3 drops with 1 spoon cold water 1 hourly 3 times daily evening for 3 days.

Frequent exposure to X-Ray is injurious to health.

Urinary system

Urine escapes on coughing.	: **Causticum 30** 2 drops with 1 spoon cold water 1 hourly 4 times a day.
Cutting pain in bladder or urethra.	: **Berberis Vulgaris Q** 6 drops with 3 spoon cold water 3 hourly 3 times daily till recovery.
Severe pain in Kidney and ineffectual desire to pass urine.	: **Nux Vom. 30** 3 drops with 1 spoon cold cold water 3 hourly 3 times daily for 5 days.
Severe backache relieved by passing urine.	: **Lycopodium 6/30** 3 drops with 1 spoon cold water 1 hourly 4 times daily for 2 days.
Severe pain in left Kidney or Ureter.	: **Hedcoma 30** 2 drops with 1 spoon cold water half hourly 3 times a day.
Severe pain in right Kidney or Ureter.	: **Lycopodium 30** 2 drops with 1 spoon cold water half hourly 3 times a day.
Reduced urination with rapid heart beats	: **Adonis Vernalis Q** 5 drops with a cup of cold water 6 hourly 2 times daily for 3 days.
Prostate enlargement	: **Hydrenja Q** 6 drops with a cup of cold water twice daily at morning and evening for 7 days.

Today's relglegency : Repentation for tomorrow.

Urinary system

Glucose in urine (Diabetes)	: **Syzizium Jamb. Q** 6 drops with a cup of cold water 4 hourly 3 times daily for 15 days.
Diabetes with Enuresis	: **Rhus Aromatica. Q** 5 drops with a cup of cold water twice daily at morning and evening for 15 days.
Urine highly coloured with pungent urinous odour	: **Benzoic Acid 30** 2 drops with 1 spoon cold water 3 hourly 3 times daily for 4 days.
Sediments in Urine	: **Lycopodium 200** 2 drops with 1 spoon cold water 3 hourly 3 times daily for 5 days.
Urine dark and scanty	: **Bryonia 200** 2 drops with 1 spoon cold water 1 hourly 3 times daily for 3 days.
Red coloured urine (Haematuria)	: **Cantharis 3x** 4 drops with 1 spoon cold water half hourly 4 times daily till recovery.
Yellow coloured urine (in Jaundice)	: **Myrica 30** 3 drops with 1 spoon cold for 7 days.
Light yellow coloured urine	: **Chelidonium 30** 3 drops with 1 spoon cold water 3 hourly 3 times daily for 3 days.

Natural food is vital food.

Urinary system

Milky Urine	: **Aurum Met. 6x** 4 drops with 1 spoon cold water 3 hourly 3 times daily till recovery.
Foamy Urine	: **Phosphoric Acid. 3x** 4 drops with 1 spoon cold water 2 hourly 2 times daily for 3 days.
Black Urine	: **Helleborous Niger 30** 3 drops with 1 spoon cold water 1 hourly 4 times daily till recovery.
Urine with sediments	: **Lycopodium 6** 3 drops with 1 spoon cold water 3 hourly 3 times daily for 7 days.
High Specific gravity in Urine	: **Syzizium Jamb. Q** 6 drops with 1 spoon cold water 6 hourly twice daily at morning and evening for 5 days.
Pus like yellow discharge with urine.	: **Cannabis Sativa 6x** 3 drops with 1 spoon cold water 3 hourly 3 times daily for 7 days.
Oedematus swelling of body with suppressed urine (Nephritis)	: **Apis Mel. 6** 4 drops with 1 spoon cold water 3 hourly 3 times daily for 10 days.

Ensure periodical urine test.

Urinary system

Frequent urination : **Gelesemium 30**
3 drops with a spoonful cold water 2 hourly 3 times daily for 3 days.

■■

> The persons having Kidney trouble of any kind should not take Coconut as it contains high grade potassium level.

Ill health invites various diseases.

LEGS

The extremities are divided into two sections i.e. Upper and Lower. The upper extremities include the limbs of hand and the lower extremities include the hip, thigh, legs, ankles, foot and toe.

The Leg (pelvic girdle to toe) is composed of various bones including the following :

1. **Femur** (thigh bone which is connected with the deep socket of the hip bone).
2. **Patella** (an additional bone known as Sesamoid Bone which is developed from a tendon and act as knee cap).
3. **Tibia and Fibula** (two different bones from knee joints to ankle. Tibia, the strong bone at the inner side i.e. on the big toe side and Fibula, the supporting bone of the Tibia is located laterally).
4. **Tarsal and Metatarsal Bones** (the tarsal bones are associated with the ankle, foot and heel (this part is known as Calcaneus). The Tarsal bones are 7 in number. The Metatarsal bones are 5 in number (in the form of a frame work of the instep).

Ensure foot care.

5. **Phalanges** (toe bones which are composed of 14 phalanges in each foot. A thick fluid known as Synovial helps folding of the bone joints).

Different muscular systems therefore carryout various movement of entire leg (thigh to toe). The following are the leg muscles attached with Tendons which initiates various movements.

1. Gluteus Maximus Muscle (helps while running and walking).
2. Gluteus Medium Muscle (helps to press the thigh together)
3. Abductor Muscle (helps to abduct the thigh)
4. Sartorius Muscle (helps to seat crosslegged)
5. Quadriceps Femoris Muscle (helps to kick)
6. Hamstring Muscles (helps in kneeling position)
7. Gastrocnemius muscle (helps to stand on tiptoe)
8. Tibialis Anterior Muscle (helps to stand on heels)
9. Flexor Digitorum Muscle (helps in movements of foot and toe).

For maintenance of blood circulation in entire leg (thigh to toe), there is a network of 10 principal arteries and 8 principal veins as mentiond below :

Arteries : External Iliac, Femoral, Deep Femoral, Popliteal Genicular, Anterior Tibial, Posterior Tibial, Posterior Tibial, Peroneal, Dorsalis, Pedis, Dorsal Metatarsal.

Veins : External, iliac, Femoral, Saphenous, Popliteal, Tibial, Venous Arch, Dorsal Digitals.

Neglegency carry risk.

Leg

The following Minerals/Vitamins are necessary for proper maintenance of systems in entire leg.

Minerals : Potassium (Fruits)
Calcium (Milk, milk products, Eggs, Green leaf, vegetables, Banana).
Phosphorus (Cereals, Pulses, Milk, Banana)
Magnesium (Green leaves, Cereals).
Vitamins : Pantothenic Acid (Yeast, Liver , Eggs)
Ascorbic Acid (Critrus fruits, Green Vegetables)
B_{12} (Meat, Fish)
D (Fish, Liver, Oil, Milk and exposure to Sun).

More importance should be given while selecting footwear. It must be comfortable, made of hygenic materials. Wearing of ill-fitting shoes may develop blisters, corns in the foot or sole, pain in thigh, cramps in culf muscle, pain and crack in heels, burning in toe. For foot care, wearing cotton socks is also advisable. Moreover, walking barefooted on grass and clean ground daily for atleast half an hour is also advisable for maintaining contact with earth which is necessary to get rid of tiredness of foot and leg.

Virtually the foot carry the weight of entire body. The ailments like sprain in ankle, knee joints, heels, sciatic pain, sore heel etc. are very common which causes great anxiety and sufferings.

The following Homoeopathic medicines are found effective for various treatments relating to leg.

Eat sufficient green vegetables.

Burning in Sole	: **Sulphur 30** 3 drops with a spoon of cold water 4 hourly 3 times daily for 3 days.
Burning feet	: **Calcarea Carb. 6** 3 drops with 1 spoon cold water once at morning daily for 10 days.
Oedematus swelling of foot	: **Iodium 30** 3 drops with one spoon cold water 3 hourly 3 times daily for 5 days.
Lameness after sprain	: **Ruta G. 200** One drop with half spoon cold water 3 hourly 4 times daily for 5 days.
Cramps in leg muscles	: **Cuprum Met. 200** 2 drops with 1 spoon cold water 3 hourly 3 times daily for 2 days.
Sore heel from rubbing of shoe.	: **Allium Cepa 30** 3 drops with a spoon cold water 2 hourly 3 times daily for 3 days.
Pain in big toe	: **Ledum Pal. 30** 2 drops with half spoon cold water 3 hourly 3 times daily for 2 days.
Deformed nails	: **Antim Crud. 200** One drop with half spoon cold water once at morning daily for 10 days.

Ensure balanced diet.

Leg

Stiffness of muscles	: **Cuprum Met. 200** 2 drops with half spoon cold water 3 hourly 3 times daily for 2 days.
Pain in bone joints	: **Ruta G.200** One drop with half spoon cold water 3 hourly 3 times daily for 7 days.
Sciatic Pain	: **Bryonia Alb. 200** 2 drops with 1 spoon cold water 6 hourly 2 times daily for 7 days.
Pain in deep muscles of leg	: **Causticum 200** 2 drops with 1 spoon cold water 3 hourly 3 times daily for 3 days.
Foot sore	: **Baryta Carb.30.** 3 drops with 1 spoon cold water 6 hourly 2 times daily for 5 days.
Sensitive corn in foot	: **Antim.Crud.200** 3 drops with 1 spoon cold water once at morning daily for 10 days.
Pain in knee joints	: **Calcarea Carb.30.** 2 drops with half spoon cold water 3 hourly 3 times daily for 10 days.
Pain from straining the flexor tondon	: **Ruta G.200.** 2 drops with 1 spoon cold water 3 hourly 4 times daily for 2 days.

Good health is the noblest gift of God.

Twitching of toe	: **Cuprum met. 200** 2 drops with half spoon cold water 2 hourly 2 times daily for 3 days.
Contraction of muscles	: **Causticum 200** 1 drop with half spoon cold water 3 hourly 3 times daily for 3 days.
Motor paralysis of muscular system.	: **Gelsemium 30.** 3 drops with 1 spoon cold water 2 hourly 3 times daily for 5 days.
Offensive foot sweat	: **Baryta carb.30.** 3 drops with a spoonful cold water once at morning daily for 10 days.

Vegetarian food is easily digestable

HEALTH GUIDE

Food is the source of nutrition. All living beings are in need of nutritious food, treated water and pollution free air to stay alive. The required amount of nutrients for a person depends on sex, age, state of health and activity. Each nurtient has specific uses in the body. The process of digestion and absorpton (see abdomen chapter) conduct supply of the following nutrients to the body cells.

1. **Carbohydrates** are the main source of energy which contains Carbon, Hydrogen and Oxygen.

Sources : Rice, Wheat, Maize, Cereals, Banana, Sugarcane, sugar etc.

2. **Protein** forms the most important constituent of our diet. It contains Nitrogen in addition to Carbon, Hydrogen and Oxygen. Proteins are Polymers (consists of 20 number of Amino Acids) which help in the break down and synthesis of Carbohydrates, Proteins and Fats.

Protein is necessary for transportation of Oxygen for respiratory system, repairing of tissues damaged during wear and tear, maintaining the healthy and active condition of muscles, skin, hair, nails. Protein act as a source of energy during starvation. Haemoglobin of blood is protein.

Sources : Pulses, Nuts, dry fruits, Meat, Eggs.

3. **Fat** constitute a major source of energy and contain less Oxygen that Carbohydrate carry. Fats produce more energy when oxidized (burnt) and also stored for consumption when necessary in the body.

Sources : Ghee, Butter, Oil, Milk, Nuts etc.

4. **Vitamins** are named as A B C D E & K. These are the substances needed in small quantity for maintaining healthy condition of bones, skin, gums, tooth, body growth and other biological functions in the body (see page 121).

Vitamin C is an important component of all the body organs. It is required for utilization of Folic acid and absorption of Iron in the body system. Vitamin C is needed for Cell respiration and to produce vital substances for Nerves, Brain and Reproductive organs. It also produces anti-stress hormones because of its highest concentration in the Adrenal glands. A protein substance 'Collagen' holds together skin cells and bone. The necessary amount of Collagen is produced by Vitamin C only. It is necessary for normal immune responses to resist infection and to aid healing of wound.

Vitamin C is not only important for maintenance of day to day health, but also in the prevention of the following diseases :

Asthma, Atherosclerosis (narrowing of the Arteries), Muscular cramps, Cancer of the Stomach, Oesophagus, Oral cavity.

Sources : Fresh citrus fruits, Lemon, Oranges, Gooseberries, Guava etc.

5. **Minerals** are inorganic salts (compound that are not Carbon based) required for metabolism and Physiological functions. The salts are ; Sodium, Calcium, Potas-

sium, Iodine, Zinc, Fluorine, Phosphorus and Iron (see page...122).

The mineral salts are needed in small quantities but they are essential for proper functioning of heart, blood, nervous system, energy currency of the body cells.

Sources : Cereal, Pulses, Milk, Butter milk, Green vegetables, common salt, Meat,fish, Water, Heeng (Asafoetida) etc.

6. **Water** : Two third of the human body consists of water alone. It is necessary for biological process in the body. It helps digestion of the food, transport of nutrients and other materials for body system and fluid balance.

Food is nothing but a natural demand of body to meet the basic need and the hunger is a silent signal. A new born baby who is ignorant about the utility, taste and required amount of food, keeps quiet when the stomach is filled. Otherwise the baby starts crying which is a signal of hunger. To meet the biological demand,they start sucking the mother's breast inquest of food i.e.milk. Virtually, a life begins with natural feeding. A child is reared up with great care and belief with need based easily digestable food items. But food habit changes during adolescence according to individual choice. Young people start eating indiscriminately due to various reasons. Over eating is the prime cause of developing stomach disorders. Hence food has to be taken in the right spirit with right consciousness. Because a low diet is simultaneously harmful for health due to depletion of minerals and vitamins.Therefore a balanced diet is absolutely necessary for all to keep the body and mind active. There should be a gap of minimum 8 hours between the two principal meals (lunch and dinner) and only light and liquid food is to be taken between the principal meals. Natural sweets like honey, sugar cane juice, fruit juice supply more energy instantly to the body cells.

To enjoy a good health , the food should be simple, pleasant, nourishing and free from chemicals, preservative, artificial colour, sedative. While eating, only half of the stomach should be filled by food and one quarter with water. The remaining quarter should be left empty. Food should not be taken when in angry mood, nervous, tense or hurry. Food should be taken in a clean, pleasant surroundings and among pleasant people.

Fresh food is the best food. Cooked long time before and preserved in refrigerator loses the food value. All seasonal fruits provide minerals and vitamins. Fasting once in a month is good for health.

■■

VITAMINS

Vitamins	Source	Function	Deficiency diseases
A (RETINOL)	Spinach, carrots, Butter, sweet-potatoes, Mango, Yellow vegetables, Fish, liver oil.	Required for healthy eyes, hair, and skin.	Poor vision, night blindness, hairfall, rough skin.
B1 (THIAMIN)	Eggs, meat, whole cereals, yeast.	Required for digestive system and regulates nervous system.	Disease called Beri-beri, extreme weakness, nervous debility.
B 2 (RIBOFLABIN)	Green leafy vegetables, peas, milk, eggs, kidney, liver.	Needed for enzyme system, oxydation of carbohydrate & Proteins.	Retarded growth, rough skin, erruption inside mouth.
B 12 (CYANOCOBALAMIN)	Meat, liver, eggs, fish.	Needed for production of blood cells and proper growth of body.	Anaemia-defficiency of red blood cells (Haemoglobin).
C (ASCORBIC ACID)	Fresh citrus fruits, lemon, oranges, Gooseberries, guava banana.	Maintains healthy skin, synthesis of Collagen, resists infection, helps to keep tooth, gum and joints healthy.	Disease called-Scurvy-swollen gum, livid spots, loose tooth and weakness in joints.
D (CALCIFEROL)	Fish, liver oil, milk and exposure to sun light.	Aids in the normal growth of bones in the young, prevents rickets.	Disease called Rickets-soft bones, spine and bow legs.
K	Green leafy vegetables, eggs, yolk.	Help in clotting of blood.	Excessive bleeding after injury.
E	All foods	Normal nutrition and defficiency problems etc. not established so far regarding Vitamin E.	

MINERALS

Minerals	Source	Functions	Deficiency diseases
CALCIUM	Milk,butter milk, green leafy vegetables, banana.	Builds bone and tooth. Regulates Heart & Muscles, nervous system,blood clotting.	Brittle bones,irregular heart beats, improper muscle movement, excessive bleeding.
PHOSPHORUS	Cereals, pulses,milk, eggs, banana.	Energy currency of body cells, builds bones and tooth.	General debility, weak tooth and bones.
IRON	Cereal, pulses, green leafy vegetables, Heeng, banana, mango, meat, prawns.	Helps transport Oxygen to blood cells and remove Carbon dioxide.	Anaemia (loss of Haemoglobin)
MAGNESIUM	Green leafy vegetables,cereals	Regulates muscle and nerves, catalyst for enzymes	Week functions of muscles and nerves
SULPHUR	Cereals, Pulses	Formation of proteins, enzymes vitamins	-do-
COBALT	Animal products	Blood cell production and synthesis of insulin.	General debility & diabetes
COPPER	Cereals, pulses, vegetables, nuts, meat, liver, fish.	Oxidation of Vitamin C and Iron, formation of Haemoglobin.	Loss of appetite,retarded growth, anaemia.
SODIUM	Common salt,most foods, coconut.	Maintenance of body fluids.	Dehydration,weakness,
POTASSIUM	Coconuts and othere foods.	Regulates the muscular and nervous system.	Nervous debility,Muscular cramps.
ZINC	Many foods	Carbon dioxide metabolism	Respiratory problems.
FLUORINE	Drinks, water, Milk.	Helps in enamel formation.	Tooth decay

Height/ Weight Guide

(Adopted from Asian Health & Diet Plan '85)

Height		Weight	
Inches	C.M.	Men	Women
4.10 "	147.3	-	44- 49 Kgs.
4.11 "	149.8	-	44- 50 Kgs.
5.0 "	152.4	-	46- 51 Kgs.
5.1 "	154.9	-	47- 53 Kgs.
5.2 "	157.5	54- 59 Kgs.	49 - 54 Kgs.
5.3 "	160.0	55- 60 Kgs	50 - 55 Kgs.
5.4 "	162.6	56- 62 Kgs.	51 - 57 Kgs.
5.5 "	165.1	58- 63 Kgs.	53 - 59 Kgs.
5.6 "	167.6	59- 65 Kgs.	54 - 61 Kgs.
5.7 "	170.2	61- 67 Kgs.	56 - 63 Kgs.
5.8 "	172.7	63- 69 Kgs.	58 - 65 Kgs.
5.9 "	175.3	64- 70 Kgs.	60 - 67 Kgs.
5.10 "	177.8	66- 73 Kgs.	62 - 69 Kgs.
5.11 "	180.3	68- 75 Kgs.	64 - 70 Kgs.
6.0 "	182.9	70- 77 Kgs.	65 - 72 Kgs.
6.1 "	185.4	72- 79 Kgs.	-
6.2 "	188.0	74- 82 Kgs.	-
6.3 "	190.5	75- 84 Kgs.	-
6.4 "	193.0	78- 86 Kgs.	-

AN AVERAGE COMPOSITION OF BALANCED DIET

Vegetarian

Sources	Average daily need		
	Food (Gr.)	Calories (Kcal)	Protein (Gr.)
Cereals	355 gr.	1150 Kcal	29 gr.
Dal & Nuts	100 gr.	320 "	22 gr.
Milk	200 ml.	235 "	8 gr.
Root Veg.	150 gr.	145 "	2 gr.
Leafy veg.	100 gr.	50 "	3 gr.
Other veg.	100 gr.	50 "	3 gr.
Fruits	100 gr.	80 "	..
Fat	50 gr.	450 "	..
Sugar or Jaggery	30 gr.	120 "	..
	Total	**2600 K.cal**	**67 gr.**

Non Vegetarian

Sources	Average daily need		
	Food (Gr.)	Calories (Kcal)	Protein (Gr.)
Cereals	355 gr.	1150 Kcal	29 gr.
Dal & Nuts	50 gr.	160 "	11 gr.
Milk	100 ml.	115 "	4 gr.
Root & Veg.	150 gr.	145 "	2 gr.
Leafy veg.	100 gr.	50 "	3 gr.
Other veg.	100 gr.	50 "	3 gr.
Fruits	100 gr.	80 "	..
Eggs	50 gr.	85 "	5 gr.
Meat/Fish	100 gr.	195 "	10 gr.
Fat	50 gr.	450 "	..
Sugar or Jaggery	30 gr.	120 "	..
	Total	**2600 K.cal**	**67 gr.**

DIET CHART WITH A LIMIT OF HIGHEST CALORIC VALUE OF FOOD ITEMS FOR DIABETICS

NON VEGETARIAN   LIMIT - 1800 K.Cal.

Diet Schedule	Food items	Quantity	Caloric Value	Total
BREAKFAST (285 K.Cal)	Tea/Coffee	1 cup	55	
	Egg (boiled)	1 pc.	80	
	Chapati with Ghee	1 pc.	150	+285 K.Cal
MID MORNING (75 K.Cal)	Apple	1 pc .(30 gr.)	25	
	Banana	1 pc.	50	+75 "
LUNCH (670 K.Cal)	Ghee	2 tsp	90	
	Rice	1 Katori	80	
	Chapati (Roti)	2 pcs.	160	
	Dal	1 katori	80	
	Chicken	50 gr	80	
	Curd	1 Cup	80	
	Vegetables	52 gr.	50	
	Banana	1 pc.	50	+670 "
EVENING TEA (135 K. Cal.)	Tea/Coffee	1 cup	55	
	Salted biscuit	6 p	80	+135 "
DINNER (535 K.Cal)	Chapati with Ghee	2 pcs	300	
	Fish	1 pc	80	
	Vegetables	78 gr.	75	
	Dal	1 Katori	80	+535 "
BED TIME (100 k.Cal.)	Milk	1 cup	100	+100 " =1800 "

DIET CHART WITH A LIMIT OF HIGHEST CALORIC VALUE OF FOOD ITEMS FOR DIABETICS

VEGETARIAN		LIMIT - 1800	K.Cal.	
Diet Schedule	Food items	Quantity	Caloric Value	Total
BREAKFAST (285 K.Cal)	Tea/Coffee	1 cup	55	
	Channa (Panir)	30 gr.	80	
	Chapati with Ghee	1 pc.	150	+285 K.Cal
MID MORNING (75 K.Cal)	Apple	1 pc .(30 gr.)	25	
	Banana	1 pc.	50	+75 "
LUNCH (670 K.Cal)	Ghee	2 tsp	90	
	Rice	1 Katori	80	
	Chapati (Roti)	2 pcs.	160	
	Dal	1 katori	80	
	Curd	1 Cup	80	
	Vegetables	135 gr.	130	
	Banana	1 pc.	50	+670 "
EVENING TEA (135 K. Cal.)	Tea/Coffee	1 cup	55	
	Salted biscuit	6 pcs	80	+135 "
DINNER (535 K.Cal)	Chapati with Ghee	2 pcs	300	
	Cheese	1 cube	80	
	vegetables	78 gr.	75	
	Dal	1 Katori	80	+535 "
BED TIME (100 k.Cal.)	Milk	1 cup	100	+100 " =1800 "

Aims which every physician should keep in mind

1. The Physician's high and only mission is to restore the sick to health.

2. The highest ideal of Cure is rapid, gentle and permanent restoration of the health or removal and annihilation of the disease in its whole extent, in the shortest, most reliable and most harmless way, on easily comprehensible principles.

Dr. SAMUEL HAHNEMANN